CAUTIOUSLY PESSIMISTIC

DEBBIE MCGEE

CAUTIOUSLY PESSIMISTIC

DEBBIE MCGEE

BREAKWATER
P.O. Box 2188, St. John's, NL   Canada   A1C 6E6
WWW.BREAKWATERBOOKS.COM

ISBN   9781778530579; 9781778530586 (ePUB)
         A CIP catalogue record for this book is available from
         Library and Archives Canada.

ILLUSTRATIONS & POSTERS
Gerry Porter except page 142 *Gerrypalooza Poster*, 2016 by Beth Oberholtzer.

PHOTOGRAPHS
page 174 *Debbie and Gerry*, 1980s by Dominique Gusset; page 202 *The Cards Guys*
& page 254 *Debbie and Gerry at Gerrypalooza* by Victoria Wells; page 246 *Debbie
and Gerry*, October 2016 by Paul Pope; page 257 Author Photo by LVImagery.

COVER ILLUSTRATION & BOOK DESIGN
Beth Oberholtzer, Oberholtzer Design Inc.

We acknowledge the support of the Canada Council for the Arts.
We acknowledge the financial support of the Government of Canada through
the Department of Heritage and the Government of Newfoundland and
Labrador through the Department of Tourism, Culture, Arts and Recreation
for our publishing activities.

PRINTED AND BOUND IN CANADA.

Breakwater Books is committed to choosing papers and materials for our books
that help to protect our environment. This book is printed on paper made of
material from well-managed forest and other controlled sources that are certified
by the Forest Stewardship Council®.

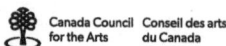
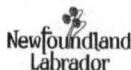

For us

Dear Reader

A selection of Gerry Porter's artwork has been included throughout this book. Some items contextualize the chapters near where they appear. Some offer insight to his personality and sense of humour. Others simply reflect his talent. To view Gerry's body of work, including his Twitter archive, please visit gporter.net.

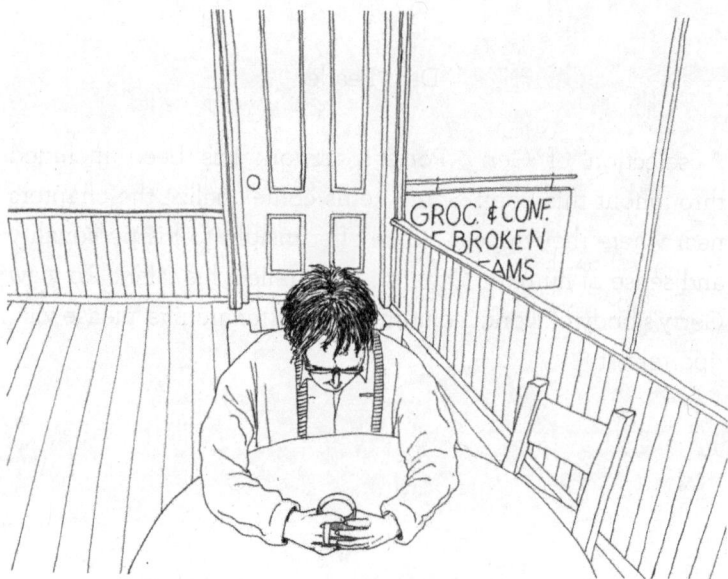

ONE

On Monday, March 28, 2016, I posted on Gerry Porter's Facebook page:

Gerry Porter

March 28, 2016

This is Gerry's wife, Debbie. What happened is that a large mass was discovered in Gerry's right temporal lobe in the wee morning hours on Easter Sunday. And it was promptly removed Monday morning. So as you can imagine, Gerry is on complete bedrest in the neurology special unit. We don't have much information on his prognosis yet, but unfortunately one of his surgeons is pretty sure cancer is involved. I will keep you updated until Gerry can use his phone again—in the meantime, he has really appreciated all of you showing your concern and affection. So keep that up, and we will post when non-family members can visit.

Three weeks earlier, I had returned to St. John's from a short visit to Mexico. I had arrived home to find the living room floor strewn with our grandkids' toys. Puzzle pieces and colourful stuffed animals trailed down the hall to the kitchen, where unwashed pots and dishes were piled on the counter. Usually, when one of us was away, the other vacuumed and dusted to have the house tidy for their return. Hmm.

The next day while out grocery shopping, Gerry stopped the car at a green light. A horn blast from behind startled him. As we moved through the intersection, he defended himself, "You can't be too careful; St. John's drivers are terrible."

"Well, that may be true," I said, "but you were the one who stopped at a green light."

I wondered if Gerry could be developing Alzheimer's, which ran in his family. He was still working full-time, but I had retired two years earlier, and I was leaving again in a week. My sister Gail was having knee replacement surgery, and I was to be her support system. I didn't discuss my concerns with anyone, but I hired a housecleaner and went on to Ottawa, where the majority of my six siblings live.

Ten days later, I was reading in bed in Ottawa, Gail and her new knee safely down for the night. It was Good Friday, March 25, 2016. My daughter-in-law Maggie texted me from a bar in St. John's, where she and my son Chris, both twenty-five-year-old musicians, were waiting to go on stage:

March 25, 2016, 11:15 p.m.

—Hey, Deb. We tried to FaceTime earlier—hoping to chat with you tomorrow sometime maybe. We are worried about Gerry.

—His memory?

—He just got pulled over by the cops for driving in the
wrong lane. Which he also did last night.

—Oh no. He was driving weird before I left. Stopped at a
green light at a busy intersection and went through a red
light on the way to the airport. I was thinking of telling you,
but I thought if it was real, you would notice it, and now
you have.

—And he got lost trying to find Gower Street. And slept
through babysitting this morning.

—He didn't wake up to babysit? He forgot? I'm not sure
he should have Jack in the car anymore.

—Yeah, we just noticed for the first time yesterday, and
it's, like, a lot all at once now. No definitely not.

—Hmm. How should we handle this? He is going to
be super-defensive. I think it is either early Alzheimer's or
cognitive impairment because of lack of sleep
and drinking.

—Jesus. He definitely doesn't get enough
sleep—may have sleep apnea.

—Yeah, the good thing about the police is it's a fact.
He can't deny it happened. The first step is for him to see
the family doctor.

—And in the meantime maybe he could take a week off
work. He slept through work yesterday too.

—You mean he missed going to work?

—Yep.

—Do you think you and Chris could sit down and talk with him about this?

—I'll talk to Chris about it after the gig. I'm certainly comfortable maybe also asking Lisa to talk to me first.

—Yes, I was thinking about Lisa too.

In the morning, I explained the situation to Gail, and we waited for a report. My cellphone rang. It was our electrician in Heart's Content, Newfoundland, inquiring if Gerry or I were coming out to meet him.

"Well, not me," I explained. "I'm in Ottawa. And Gerry doesn't seem to be well, so we might have to make another arrangement."

"I wondered," he replied, and told me that Gerry had phoned him at two a.m. on Thursday night. My heart dropped. This was getting worse and worse. It was time for Lisa, Gerry's sister.

Maggie was on it.

March 26, 2016, 1:36 p.m.

—Okay, Lisa's on her way in from Ochre Pit Cove. We're going to try to get Gerry to go to the hospital today.

— What a relief! I'm feeling very teary.

—Chris just got to your house. Gerry's still asleep. Wearing his pjs. Sound system was blasting. Wearing his glasses with the iPad on his chest. Groceries not put away, on the kitchen floor. Freya had no food.

—I'm scared—so glad you two are on the case. Maybe it's a
series of little strokes.

—Could be anything. Gerry's supposed to be hosting
poker tonight.

—I'll call Ed and tell him poker will need to be changed.

I assisted Gail to a chair in the living room, put ice on her
swollen knee, and sped to the nearest store to purchase a
turkey breast and trimmings for tomorrow's Easter dinner. We
settled down to wait, speculating uneasily on what could be
wrong with Gerry. At last there was news from Maggie.

March 26, 2016, 4:52 p.m.

—Okay, he's on the way to the hospital now.

—Fantastic! Who is with him?

—Lisa and Chris, and I'll meet them there later.

—Okay, I'll find out more later. I'm so relieved—it's a
start. Thank you so much.

—♡

I texted Lisa to thank her for looking after Gerry.

March 26, 2016, 5:15 p.m.

—How does he seem to you?

—He's not himself. He can converse fine, but had a hard
time with his shoelaces.

—I'm pretty scared.

—We'll figure it out. He's chatting normally.

There was nothing to do but wait. To distract ourselves, Gail and I ate popcorn and chocolate bunnies while watching the second season of the tense British thriller *Happy Valley* on the living room television. I felt guilty for being in such comfort, while those on the front lines sat on cold plastic seats in a crowded ER, no doubt reading their phones. But I also had a sense that they had enough to deal with without constant interrogation from me. I tried to restrain myself, but after two episodes, I checked in with Maggie.

March 26, 2016, 9:32 p.m.

—Any news?

—Nope. Still waiting to be seen. They are in Overload
   Capacity Protocol.

—I'm so sorry, it must be hellish.

—Gerry is in good spirits. He wanted us to go unlock the
   door at the house so everyone could go to poker.

—He must be freaked out. I texted to ask what he was up to,
   he just said it's a long story, I'll catch you up later. Do you
   think he knows I'm aware of the situation?

—We haven't mentioned you. He doesn't know much.
   We've been very quiet.

—Okay, let's leave it like that. I told Nick. Spoke to him on the
   phone. He's upset, of course.

—Gerry is in with the Dr now for the last half-hour . . .

. . . Okay, he's getting a CT scan. Lisa is staying with him, and we're going home.

We finished all six episodes, and still no news. Exhausted, I assisted Gail to bed and fretted myself to sleep, checking my phone as soon as I awoke. Lisa had left a text at four a.m., asking me to call when I was up.

Damn, that did not sound positive. And if she had been up at four in the morning, I wasn't going to call her. I was assembling Gail's breakfast of yoghurt and toast when Maggie phoned.

I watched a blueberry on the kitchen floor as she told me the CT had revealed a mass in Gerry's right temporal lobe. "Lisa said the tumour was so large the doctors couldn't believe he walked in on his own."

He had immediately been admitted to the neurology floor and was scheduled for surgery tomorrow.

"I'll try and get a flight today," I told her. "Talk soon." I picked up the blueberry.

Gail, who had been sipping coffee and watching my face as the conversation unfolded, sounded unsurprised when I told her our worst fears were realized. "He has a tumour and is going to have brain surgery."

I had to get home. I had to find someone to look after Gail. I had to tell Nick, our twenty-eight-year-old son going to school in Toronto. I was receiving phone calls from the hospital, asking for my consent to operate. Because it was Easter Sunday, nephews and nieces dropped in to visit. I packed through the chaos, and my brother Jim came to pick me up.

"We lost Mom in 2014, Dad in 2015, and I won't be able to handle losing Gerry in 2016," I said as we neared the airport, my voice thickening.

"He's not going to die," Jim replied soothingly.

In the St. John's airport, I gazed at the bottom of the arrivals' escalator. Gerry had always been there to get me when I came home. Instead, Chris and Maggie were there. They delivered me straight to the Health Sciences Centre. It was 11:30 p.m. Nick had arrived an hour before me, Gerry's dad would arrive an hour later.

I found Gerry ensconced in a four-person ward, with an in-room nursing station staffed with two nurses. This level of care impressed upon me even further the seriousness of the situation. Gerry was sitting up in bed, wearing his own pyjamas, and I bent over to kiss him, saying, "Well, you've been busy!" He smiled back at me, looked over at Nick, and said, "Everybody's here!"

I felt a mixture of things—relieved to be there, anxious about tomorrow, and kind of like a spectator. Lisa, Chris, and Maggie were in charge. Nick, Gerry's dad, and I were like bit players, in need of direction. Gerry's father would stay at Lisa's. I wondered what would be waiting for Nick and me at home.

Three monitors were beeping quietly, the nurse kept checking his vitals, and Gerry seemed rather pleased by all the attention. Poker and work friends had been dropping in to visit all day. But now, with only his closest family present, Gerry didn't say much. He kept checking his phone, even looking at it over his father's shoulder when they were hugging hello. I got the sense his phone was grounding him. Around one a.m., the nurse ushered us out. Visiting hours were long over, and it would be a big day tomorrow.

At seven the next morning, we gathered again in Gerry's room. This time he was wearing a blue hospital gown and was on a wheeled stretcher. "Look after it," he said, handing me his phone. Joking and laughing, the gang of us accompanied Gerry like a mobile comedy club, as the good-natured orderly pushed his stretcher along the antiseptic hallway to the elevator. There were six of us, plus the orderly and Gerry, and when the elevator doors opened at each of the four floors on the way down, we smiled appreciatively at the waiting passengers who shook their heads. The surgical unit was right across from the elevator. Were we really going to let this happen? Just as Gerry was about to disappear behind the doors marked "surgery," Chris darted over, stopping the forward momentum. He bent over to rest his head on Gerry's chest for one last hug. "I love you, Dad." And then Gerry was gone, the doors swinging closed behind him.

We shuffled our feet like a small herd of cattle, unsure what to do next. A nurse in surgical scrubs herded us to a small waiting room for relatives of patients in surgery. "It will be at least a few hours," she said. "We'll come and get you when he's out." The room was welcoming, with sun coming in the windows, and we all found a spot to nest, Lisa and her dad on a sofa, Nick and I on chairs, while Chris and Maggie went off to fill our coffee orders.

As we waited, I looked at Gerry's phone. I saw that even through the past twenty-four hectic hours, he had still managed to post on Facebook, a photo of our four-year-old grandson, Jack, sitting on his hospital bed, and of the sunrise from his hospital room window. The hospital photos had resulted in over sixty comments and questions on his Facebook page. As I sat in the waiting room, people began texting me directly, wanting to know why Gerry was in the hospital.

But now was not the time to respond. I was consumed with more pressing issues such as, would the surgery result in brain damage? Maybe I would never again have a conversation with Gerry as I knew him. Our anxiety increased as time went on. "He should be out by now," Lisa said. Nick ventured in search of an update but returned defeated, reporting, "Nobody knows anything about him." It had now been over four hours. Was he dead? I had the inspiration to phone his room. The nurse answered right away.

"This is Gerry Porter's wife. Do you know if he's still in surgery?"

"We've been wondering where you all went! He's here! They brought him up an hour ago."

We scrambled upstairs, and sure enough, he was alive and awake enough to know we were there. He was now hooked up to an IV. There was a large white bandage on the right side of his head, with tubing running out of it. I guessed it was for draining the wound. The in-room nurse had Gerry and a newly arrived roommate to look after, and we knew he would get excellent care. I spared a warm and fuzzy thought for the Canadian health care system. "He'll be on twenty-four-hour bedrest," the nurse said. "But we'll get him on his feet tomorrow."

The surgeon and the neurologist came in, speaking first to the nurse and then joining us at the bedside.

"The operation went well," said the surgeon. "We got the entire mass."

"We're pretty sure it's malignant," the neurologist added, "but we've sent it to pathology to be certain. It should take a few days to get the results."

Gerry thanked them as they left, and we all murmured assent. "No point in worrying about it yet," Gerry said. I backed him up. "Yep, one thing at a time. First order of business: heal from brain surgery." Chris, Nick, Lisa, and Gerry Sr. all nodded.

He had survived, and as he seemed to know who we were and what had happened to him, I decided he was still himself. Now I had to do something about all those questioning Facebook friends. "I guess I'll post on your Facebook," I said, and did so from his computer at home that night. The post received 149 reactions, 180 comments, and 7 shares. Each comment was heartfelt and very welcome. Gerry's friends, my friends, his sister's friends, our sons' friends, and especially our relatives—it was comforting to think they were wishing us well. I didn't know it yet, but our public journey through cancer was underway.

As promised, the next day Gerry was up and walking the hallways with the support of a physiotherapist. I posted pictures of him on Facebook, dashing in a red-and-white checked kimono, the scary tube still running from his bandaged head. That night, March 29, I posted on his Facebook:

🎧 **Gerry Porter**
March 29, 2016

Hi, friends. Gerry can have visitors starting tomorrow! Hours are 11–2, 4:30–6:30, and 8–9 p.m. Two allowed at a time, but for the time being most visits are pretty short, so you won't wait long in any case! Be gentle—his head hurts!

Soon his visitors were posting their findings. Such as:

♣ Ger is in good hands, in good spirits, and has a great view. He truly appreciates the messages sent his way. Signage in the hospital needs a bit of work.

People sent him jokes, memes, links to music and to photos they thought he might enjoy. I spent time every day poring over the comments on Facebook and diligently liking each of them, as a way of showing my appreciation for their love and concern.

An old friend of Gerry's posted:

✚ My dear Gerry . . . as an FB and real-life friend,
I feel a responsibility to turn the tables and amuse you with
a little post. I begin (inspired by your oeuvre of haiku) with
a humble limerick about your own self. Here goes:

There once was a pundit named Porter,
About whom I can say I'm a supporter,
His Facebook rants, quite intelligent,
Express a wide range of sentiments,
He might love it or leave it, drawn and quartered.

In the real world, friends were arriving on our stoop with soup, bread, tea buns, and even rabbit ragu. Between the moral support on Facebook and the physical support at the house and hospital, we felt well and truly held, cared for by our community.

But all was not well. It was no joke when I posted on April 1:

Debbie McGee
April 1, 2016

Not a good week for the McGee-Porter household. Monday,
Gerry had his brain surgery. Tuesday, Debbie (me!) fell ill with a
"stomach flu." Wednesday, everybody else carried on, but Gerry
Porter was very weak and nauseous. Thursday, Maggie
collapsed with exhaustion. So Nick held the fort at the hospital,

while Chris cared for Maggie, Gerry continued to sleep, and Lisa was everywhere at once.

Today, Friday, Gerry is feeling much better—ate food for the first time in two days and had a walk with the physio. I still have not seen him since Tuesday. Nicholas McGee has succumbed to whatever this bug is and is now struck off-strength. The wonderful Maggie Keiley just delivered us Gravol and ginger ale, to go along with our applesauce. So, friends, if you visit Gerry be sure to use hand cleanser on your way in and out of the hospital. But do go in if you can, 'cause his wife and kids have to stay away for a while. Sure hoping Lisa Porter and her dad, Gerry Porter Sr., manage to stay healthy!

Our situation felt surreal. I was not able to go back to the hospital until Saturday, April 2. Not seeing Gerry for three days made me again feel like a spectator. I made up for my absence when I returned by doing something only an intimate partner could—helping him have his first bath since surgery. By now the creepy tubing was gone, and even his white head bandage was off.

I ran hot water in the tub, which took up most of the cupboard-sized bathroom we had been assigned. It did us both good to be alone for the first time in weeks, as I soaped his hair and washed his back.

"You have no idea how good this feels," he said.

I smiled. "Oh, I dunno, I have some idea." I took a picture of his scar, so he could see it for himself. It was raised and red and looked to be held together by staples. It began near his right temple, running vertically for about four inches and then gently curving along the top of his head for another three. "I really want to get home," he said. "The food here is terrible."

After the bath, we met with the surgeons to discuss the results of the pathology report in a consulting room on the neurology floor. Gerry and I sat on one side of the table, me slightly damp, Gerry in clean pyjamas and robe. The clinical associate cleared his throat.

"The report confirms the tumour was indeed cancerous," he informed us, "a primary gliosarcoma, to be precise."

"We were expecting that," said Gerry.

We had been living with the assumption that it was cancer from the day of the surgery. Having it confirmed was not a shock.

"You'll have to be strong," the doctor said, his eyes not quite meeting mine.

That alarmed me, but not as much as when he added that since the oncologists at the Cancer Centre would determine the treatment plan, we should save our questions for them. "They will be much more helpful to you."

It must be bad, I thought. *He doesn't even want to talk to us about it.*

The good news was that Gerry would be discharged on Monday. Only a few more hospital meals to go.

I googled gliosarcoma when I went home for supper. After a few minutes, I resolved not to read any further. I would wait until we met with the oncologist and get an expert opinion. I told Gerry this when I returned to the hospital that night. "I did the same," he said. "Goodbye, Dr. Google."

Gerry's phone had been returned to him while I was off sick, and he had begun responding to friends' inquiries on Messenger and posting on Facebook.

Gerry loved using social media. His sense of humour was a perfect match for it. Always a wit with funny one-liners, he was a graphic artist genius, adept with Photoshop, able to quickly craft amusing pictures. When Facebook and Twitter came along, he had an immediate outlet and audience, especially for his memes.

He now had 1,186 friends on Facebook, 1,500 followers on Twitter, a YouTube channel, and his own blog, *Cautiously Pessimistic*. His habit was to read through news feeds and various sites on a daily basis and post anything that interested him and that he thought would interest others.

When I drove him home on April 4, after a total of nine nights in hospital, he went straight upstairs to bed. He also returned to Twitter, using his handle @ficklesonance.

**�>�
 Gerry Porter**
@ficklesonance

I deny any wrongdoing. I also deny any right doing.

9:40 AM – 4 Apr 2016

Ω replying to @ficklesonance
Hey. Good to see you back.

▫ replying to @ficklesonance
The king has returned!!

Nick, Chris, Maggie, and the little ones were still under the weather, so they had to avoid contact with Gerry for the first few days. But I notified the rest of the world.

Debbie McGee
April 4, 2016

So, Gerry Porter came home today! He is so much happier. His cancer is a primary gliosarcoma. We don't know more than that—waiting for our visit to the Cancer Centre.

Onwards and upwards! Thanks for all your support, your food, and your love. We'll keep you posted.

Within a day, Gerry was up, making himself bacon and eggs in the morning and cuddling with our cat, Freya. It was another ten days before the appointment with the medical oncologist. In the interim, our only medical appointments were at a public health clinic, first to check his head wound and later to get the Frankenstein stitches removed. They were replaced with less alarming adhesive bandage strips. We used the time to recover, to visit, and to hang out with Nick, who had to return to Toronto on April 11 to present the written comprehensive exams for his doctorate in modern Chinese history. We even went to a book launch for Gerry's best friend, Ed Riche, at The Ship Pub, where Gerry received applause just for being there. And, of course, he amused himself on Twitter.

◻◻ Gerry Porter
@ficklesonance
Maybe the Tories and NDP could consider a "Unite the Wrong" movement.
6:55 PM - 10 Apr 2016

◻◻ Gerry Porter
@ficklesonance
After the Muskrat Falls debacle comes the "Figuring out what went wrong with Muskrat Falls" debacle, so our dance card is full debacle-wise.
1:31 PM - 13 Apr 2016

At nine a.m. on April 15, three weeks after the emergency room, we had our first appointment at the Dr. H. Bliss Murphy Cancer Centre. Neither of us had been in the Cancer Centre before. It is a small, modern-looking building with a large glass atrium. I remember green plants and sunshine and being startled when a brass bell rang out as we entered the lobby. "Someone has just finished their last treatment," the receptionist explained.

The treatment area itself is reached by descending an attractive, wide staircase. There are various areas to sit downstairs, depending on whether you are coming for clinic, chemotherapy, or radiation. The atmosphere is different from the main hospital, which is right next door. All the staff are cheerful and patient—it must be a prerequisite for working there. I imagined all the nurses, technicians, and receptionists over the years who had been sent back to the main hospital after being just a little too crabby.

Also unlike the main hospital, everyone is there for the same reason. You can't always tell who the patient is and who is the support person, but mostly the pallid skin, the missing body parts, or the faltering walk gives it away. In our case, it was the shaved right side of Gerry's head and the fresh three-cornered scar.

The clinic waiting area was filled with rows of hardwood chairs, a bit like a classroom. There were several doors on the side, through which patients and doctors entered and exited. Gerry and I sat on the softest-looking chairs halfway down, pondering our questions, which I had written in a turquoise notebook recently picked up at Shoppers. I had dubbed it The Gerry Book. "I think I'll ask if they know when the cancer started," I said, adding it to the list.

Eventually, we were called to one of the side doors and found it opened to a narrow consulting room, with a back door that seemed to lead to an inner sanctum. "The doctor will be right in," said the nurse, exiting through the back door. We settled on much softer chairs and were beginning to look around us when the medical oncologist entered, carrying a file. "No, no, don't get up," she said. After introductions and hand-shakes, she too sat down.

She was thankfully direct with us.

A gliosarcoma is a lethal form of brain cancer. It is very rare, very aggressive, and hard to control. It was primary, meaning it had grown in the spot where it was found. It had probably been there for three to a maximum of six months.

As to prognosis, only 25 per cent of patients live one year. Only 10 per cent live two years. A very few had lived as long as five years.

Gerry would not return to work.

He would never drive again.

He should make sure his will was in order.

If there was anything important he needed to tell somebody, he should not put it off.

Words that you only read in novels, or hear in a play or movie, being said out loud—and to us! We were apparently expected to make sense of them. She gazed at us, gauging our reaction.

"Sounds like bucket-list time," Gerry said.

The doctor smiled, probably relieved. Even in my state of shock, I was impressed with Gerry's response.

She outlined the treatment plan: five days a week of radiation and oral chemotherapy, for six weeks. After that, oral chemo would continue monthly for a year.

We thanked her and staggered out, redeemed our parking ticket, and held hands on the way to the car park. At home, we lay on the bed and cried.

Then we composed ourselves and got on the phone to our children and relatives. Telling them was less difficult than we expected, because unlike us, they had read the information they found through Google and already knew a gliosarcoma was extremely serious.

What to tell the community? We opted for middle-ground honesty, and two days later I posted on Facebook:

Debbie McGee
April 17, 2016

So here's the update on Gerry Porter. He will start six weeks of radiation and chemotherapy, Monday to Friday, on April 25. When that finishes in early June, he will continue on with chemo on a regular basis for a year. It's an aggressive cancer, but with this treatment we are hoping for the best. Thanks for all your encouragement and support—it helps tremendously.

Gerry was now back in full form on social media, sitting in front of his computer in our shared office, creating scathing memes, including one on the closure of public libraries that was shared 1,779 times on Facebook. Many of his tweets were jokes about local politics.

Gerry Porter
@ficklesonance
It must be awkward conducting provincial cabinet meetings with all those pants on fire. #nlpoli
8:39 AM - 20 Apr 2016

We differed in our use of social media. For example, in May 2016, I posted on Facebook a total of twenty-three times. Gerry, on the other hand, shared fifty-eight links and stories and five songs, posted twenty-four pictures of family and eighteen original pieces, either written satire, photoshopped pictures or memes, or his news haikus, limericks, and found poetry that came from the comments section on news sites.

Also, I didn't use Twitter. Gerry had three accounts, tweeting as @ficklesonance (547 tweets in May), @NewfKarlMarx (23 tweets), and @harperstemper (7 tweets). Many of them were just for fun, like this one from his character NewfKarlMarx, a folksy kind-of socialist.

> **⚒ NewfKarlMarx**
> @NewfKarlMarx
> I was told to dress in layers for the cold, but frankly all these chickens make me look ridiculous.
> 9:55 AM - 20 Apr 2016

I rarely knew what Gerry was doing on his phone or computer, but when I first read his Twitter feed a year later I was not surprised to see how funny his tweets were. On Twitter, it's all about being part of the ongoing thread. If you aren't paying attention, you'll miss your chance to be witty and get the gratification and validation of likes and, even better, retweets. No wonder he had to keep his phone in his hand as we watched Netflix, checking whenever it buzzed.

I had told my family and close friends the full truth about Gerry's prognosis. Gerry had not. Lisa and her family knew the story, but he had let his father believe that the treatment would possibly cure him. His friends knew it was serious, especially if they knew how to use Google, but he did not discuss it with them.

We resolved to live our lives as normally as possible. Gerry kept a digital Evernote diary on his computer, writing just a few lines each night about the day's events. The month of May shows radiation treatment five days a week, daily oral chemotherapy, weekly blood tests, six clinic appointments, a lot of grocery shopping, cooking (on Gerry's part), many visits with friends and relatives, eight meals in restaurants, a play, another book launch, and Netflix. Lots of Netflix. We also spent several nights at our beloved country place in Heart's Content, tending to a major bathroom renovation.

For me, time was transformed. I had been a practicing Buddhist for ten years and understood the notion of being in the present moment. Still, I was surprised at my clarity and focus. I gave up my position on the Newfoundland Independent Filmmakers Co-operative (NIFCO) board of directors and stopped volunteering as a meditation instructor for Shambhala. I forgot everything I knew about history, politics, philosophy. Instead I focused on what medications had to be taken and when, what time the radiation appointments were, what chores had to be done, and whether Gerry's energy levels allowed for socializing. I think of myself as reticent, but I suddenly had no problem being direct in my pursuit of whatever was needed, especially when dealing with Gerry's long-term disability claim, a nightmare of offices, paperwork, and signatures.

Gerry was continuing with his design work, creating two posters and a T-shirt for the thirtieth anniversary of the Fleming Street Massacre, a seminal event where a noisy arts party had been raided by police. No one was hurt, but musicians, actors, students, and one New Democrat MHA had been loaded in a paddy wagon and spent the night in jail. Gerry had been there but left before the raid, and I had been in Gander. So neither of us got arrested, but everyone who had was our friend or acquaintance.

Gerry watched baseball and hockey on TV and played cards with his cherished poker buddies. He was also having fun on Twitter.

◯◯ Gerry Porter
@ficklesonance
You know, if there actually *was* a gravy train, that'd be great.
8:07 AM - 6 May 2016

Harper's Temper had been a favourite account of his during the years that Stephen Harper had been prime minister, but with the election of the Trudeau Liberals in 2015, Gerry only tweeted from it occasionally.

✹ Harper's Temper
@harperstemper
Christ. The Long Form Census. Sure then. Yeah. Ché Guevara lives here. Stalin's in the guest bedroom. Whatever, fuckers.
8:14 AM - 9 May 2016

Mixed in with his political comments, retweets of the posts of others, and general pontificating, Gerry participated in hashtag games on Twitter, where the idea is to come up with a clever twist on an element of pop culture, like this spin on movie titles:

◯◯ Gerry Porter
@ficklesonance
Tinker Tailor Soldier Pie. #MealAMovie
2:59 PM - 11 May 2016

Seventh Seal Carcass. #MealAMovie

3:56 PM - 11 May 2016

Lovage, Actually. #MealAMovie

4:01 PM - 11 May 2016

The Great Garlic Scape. #MealAMovie

4:09 PM - 11 May 2016

The Grated Dictator. #MealAMovie

4:16 PM - 11 May 2016

The Borscht Ultimatum. #MealAMovie

4:30 PM - 11 May 2016

Romaine Holiday. #MealAMovie

4:35 PM - 11 May 2016

There were many more title suggestions, but these give a sense of the fun Gerry was having. For the moment, his blood tests were good, he was just a little fatigued from the radiation treatment, and we continued to hope he would be one of the outliers and live for five years.

————

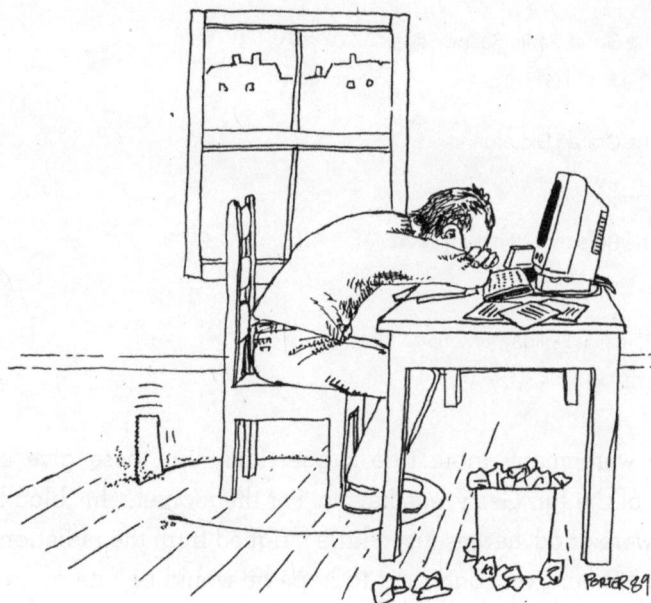

THE DESPAIR OF THE 80'S
MEETS THE IRONY OF THE 90'S.

TWO

I'm not from Newfoundland. I moved to St. John's from Vancouver on October 1, 1985. Both of my children were born in Newfoundland, and I have good street cred, so I like to think I've moved up from being a come from away. More like a landed immigrant.

I'm not from Vancouver, either. I lived there for five years, doing my master of arts in communication at Simon Fraser University and making my first film, *Little Mountain: An Election from the Inside*. Before that, I lived in Ottawa for fifteen years, and before that, Victoria, BC. My dark secret is that I was actually born in Toronto, something that does not go over well on either coast.

My first visit to St. John's was in May 1985, as a delegate to the annual general meeting of the national association of film-makers' co-operatives. The meeting was hosted by NIFCO, the Newfoundland Independent Filmmakers Co-operative. I was a member of Cineworks, the Vancouver film co-op, and delighted to get a chance to travel across the country. I only knew one person in St. John's, filmmaker Paul Pope. We were both on the board of the national association.

Paul and NIFCO put a tremendous effort into showing off St. John's to the visiting delegates. We climbed up Signal Hill, went iceberg hunting on a schooner, ate a huge baked cod in the middle of the night. We drank at The Ship and partied at the LSPU Hall (The Hall), two St. John's arts institutions. Those of us who wanted could shoot a roll of film, which was processed in the NIFCO film lab. The resulting film, *Alliance on the March*, edited and narrated by NIFCO member Mike Jones, was shown at the closing party. He'd done it in the style of a newsreel from the Second World War. So funny! My friend Cari Green and I drove "around the bay" for two nights, visiting quaint little towns whose names we consistently mispronounced.

Before Cari and I left Newfoundland, we went to the LSPU Hall to see *Out of the Bin*, a one-man show by CODCO member Andy Jones. I had seen a lot of Canadian theatre, becoming a fan when my grade ten class in Ottawa had been bussed to the brand-new National Arts Centre to see *The Ecstasy of Rita Joe*. But I had never seen anything as unique as Andy's show. By the time I returned to Vancouver, I was in love with St. John's and with the talent, energy, and creativity of not only NIFCO, but the entire arts community. I made a plan to go back.

When I returned four months later, on October 1, 1985, my initial idea was to stay in St. John's for just a few months. I needed to move on from a relationship that had ended, and I wanted to live in a fun and inspiring place while developing a documentary about the middle class, *The New Poverty*. Days before I left Vancouver, I had received a film production grant from the Canada Council for the Arts for this project. So I was in good shape when I arrived—had some money, had a project, and already had some friends.

I wrote to a friend in Vancouver, trying to describe my new life:

I'm living in The Terrace, a beautiful old house, with lots of plants, three cats, a view of the harbour, and roommates Ange and Evelyn. I connected right in with the community, and I feel more at home and less alienated than I have since leaving Ottawa. I think it is the size of the city. I live downtown, I can walk anywhere I want to go, I know a lot of people and I see them all the time, it's easy to meet people, and there are no tall buildings to tower over me. The harbour is mostly unobstructed by high-rises, and unlike Vancouver, you don't have to be rich to live next to the water. I love it.

It's quite tight, everyone hangs out in the same few places, and it's easy to meet people in other disciplines. As a result, there's this amazing cross-fertilization that makes the work going on here one notch up from any other place I've ever been. You sit around at The Ship, the local pub, and at one table there's a poet, a musician, lots of actors, filmmakers, dancers, writers, visual artists—and they're all talking to one another about their projects and feeding each other with ideas and inspiration. Of course, not everything is ideal, but I'm still new enough that the politics and intrigue doesn't affect me, cause it doesn't involve me (yet!).

Our house was known as The Terrace because it was situated at the bend of a large cul-de-sac off Gower Street known as the Masonic Terrace. Our official address was Willicott Lane. The huge Masonic Temple, constructed in 1896, backed on one side of the cul-de-sac, and heritage houses surrounded the rest. Ange and Evelyn and I lived in the upstairs of The Terrace, and our neighbour Bruce lived in a one-bedroom apartment downstairs. Attached to us was a duplicate house and apartment, owned by a professor at the university. Our side had a kitchen and living room on the first floor, as well as Ange's bedroom. On the second floor were one large, one small, and one teeny bedroom, and a bathroom with a large claw-foot bathtub and a spectacular view of St. John's Harbour. I moved into the small bedroom, which had a small arched window that looked out onto the cul-de-sac and was furnished with a double bed. The Terrace was a five-minute walk from The Hall, six minutes from The Ship, and ten minutes from NIFCO. It was perfect.

To top it off, I had auditioned for and been invited to join Sarabande, a women's singing group. The fifteen of us rehearsed on Thursday nights, finishing up afterwards at The Ship, where we stayed until the lights came on at one in the morning. The laughter! I loved St. John's.

My first memory of Gerry is from a kitchen party on Gower Street, not long after I had arrived in St. John's. The Blue Jays were in the playoffs, and we followed the game from the TV on top of the refrigerator. It was clearly an arts crowd—a poet, a photographer, an actor. Gerry was sitting at the kitchen table, next to his girlfriend, Joan, the editor of the magazine *Arts in formation*. He had longish curly hair, big wire glasses, and was thin and nervous. His feet were tapping, his hand always held a cigarette, and although he was funny, he was not my type. Or more precisely, not the type I was currently looking for.

A month or so later, I saw Gerry at a hearing for the Royal Commission on Employment and Unemployment, held in the community room of a church in the west end of St. John's. He was covering it for his job at the *Evening Telegram*, and I was there doing research for my film project. Recognizing me from downtown, he asked if I wanted to share his cab back to The Ship, courtesy of his employer. We chatted easily enough in the cab, but what I most remember is how he took off once we reached the inside of The Ship. Did he even say goodbye? Off to Joan and *Star Trek*, which they watched in the corner next to the pool table each weekday at five-thirty.

After that, I have no memories of Gerry until the early summer of 1986. By then I was pals with his good friend Ed Riche. I had put my documentary aside to help Ed produce his short film, *Roland's Progress*. Ed and Gerry and Joan shared an apartment on the corner of Victoria and Gower Streets. Joan had recently broken up with Gerry, and I remember Ed telling me what an awful situation they were all in, as Gerry pretended it didn't matter when Joan brought home her new boyfriend. According to Ed, Gerry was drinking too much. He certainly had crazy eyes whenever I saw him, mostly at The Ship. There were also rumours that he was sleeping around, lots of one-night stands, apparently something new for him.

Gerry had a role in Ed's film, which was shot in August of 1986. It was a minor part, and I mainly recall his spaced-out demeanour and that he only smiled with his mouth closed, because his front teeth were in bad shape. Gerry and Ed were now living on Alexander Street. I remember Gerry cutting my hair into a stylish mullet on their back deck prior to the shoot. He had a nice, light touch. I could tell he was interested in me.

But nothing came of it, and he seemed to have an alcohol-fuelled relationship happening with Mary, a powerhouse actor well-known in the community. I had hung out with Mary on several occasions over the past year and knew her much better than I knew Gerry. One night after a cabaret show at The Hall,

Gerry approached me as I chatted with Ed in the hallway. He suggested going to a Thomas Trio dance at the Bella Vista later that week, and I agreed that would be fun. Before we could make any plans, Mary came in and swept him away in her whirlwind.

By fall 1986, I had succumbed to the magic that was the St. John's filmmaking community and was reworking my documentary into a short drama. I worked on the script in my small upstairs bedroom at The Terrace, sitting at a table crowded with a lamp, a desk phone, an IBM PC Jr. computer, and a dot-matrix printer. My goal was to shoot the film after Christmas, so there wasn't much time to assemble a cast and crew and plan the production schedule. But I had been in St. John's for a year now and knew I would get lots of support from the film and acting community.

It was around this time that Gerry and I got together. Did we go for supper at The Curry House on Water Street? I remember meeting him there around that time and that he knew what to order. Or maybe we saw a show at The Hall. All I know for sure is that one night sitting alone on the couch in The Terrace living room, he offered to give me a back massage, something I later referred to as his patented signature move. We ended up in my crowded bedroom, where we had surprisingly good sex. Surprising, because in my experience, most men weren't very good lovers. This increased my interest in seeing him. Maybe he was my type after all.

Gerry had left his job at the newspaper and was now working as a staff writer at *Arts in formation*, in their offices above The Ship, and we began meeting for drinks after work.

I got to know a bit about him. He was twenty-four, nine years younger than me. He had been born in St. John's. His parents had split up a few years earlier, and his mother was still in the family home. Gerry was estranged from his father, who had moved to Ottawa. He had one sister, Lisa.

Gerry enjoyed local fame due to his work as a comic and cartoon artist and from his stint as editor of the student newspaper, *The Muse*. He had not finished his university degree but instead spent a year in Ottawa, as the president of Canadian University Press, a newswire service owned by student newspapers across Canada. He was now establishing himself as a writer from his work on the *Evening Telegram* and *Arts in formation* and was also using his graphic art skills to create posters, murals, and flyers for events at the LSPU Hall.

Even though he was young, his association with Mary gave him some credibility in my eyes. I had not given much thought to her relationship with Gerry, assuming it had ended, or he wouldn't be seeing me. She was currently in Halifax, working on a television series. But when she returned home about a month later, I heard she had held a party and that Gerry had been there. That was not unusual, but why had he not told me about it? My instincts told me something was up.

It was understandable if he wanted to revive a relationship with her, but I was not willing to take a back seat to someone else. So far Gerry and I had not spoken of any feelings for one another. Asking him about Mary might be admitting that I cared, which I wasn't sure I did. I had many other things to worry about, including getting up the nerve to ask Andy Jones to play a lead character in my film. Gerry came with me and stood outside in the cool fall air while I phoned Andy from a phone booth on Duckworth Street. I was elated when he accepted, and as Gerry and I walked toward The Ship, I told him I had heard about the party and asked directly if something was going on between him and Mary.

"I don't want to interfere in whatever it is, but I do want to know."

"Nothing is going on. It's over. We're just friends."

I was surprised at my relief. So no complications then.

It's a small town, and I ran into Mary the next day. We stopped for a chat. She said she hadn't known I had been seeing Gerry. I got the sense she was surprised I was bothering with him. She also said he had been at her welcome-home party all night. This was new information. I did not ask her for any details.

Had he told me the truth? I determined to find out.

That night at The Ship, Gerry and I sat by ourselves at a small table, drinking draft beer. Dire Straits' "Walk of Life" was playing. I toyed with the rim of my glass.

"Mary said you stayed at her house the night of the party."

He took a sip of his beer. "Yes."

"Did you sleep with her?"

"Yes."

I upended the table, showering him in beer. Without another word, I stormed out, slamming the door behind me. I hoped he would be humiliated, everybody staring and wondering. I also expected him to come after me, but he didn't. Later I found out that someone had picked him up, righted the table, and helped him find his glasses, which turned out to be broken.

Even I was surprised by my reaction. Now I can see that my response was not just to the immediate hurt but to the hurts of the past as well. Almost ten years earlier, I had been in a relationship with a university professor I had met during a political campaign. I adored him, but over the five years we were together, he had lied and cheated and gaslighted, and by the time I left him, I did not have much trust in men.

Gerry had just confirmed the wisdom of that position. I had made myself vulnerable enough to ask about him and Mary, and he lied. Or at least omitted something I had the right to know. Why couldn't he have just told me the truth when I asked the first time? It would not have been a deal-breaker. Now I wasn't sure what to do.

I knew from my conversation with Mary that she didn't see Gerry as a suitable long-term partner for herself. And Gerry had told me it was over between them. But I still wanted him, physically at least. I wasn't so angry I couldn't sleep with him. I called Gerry a few days later, and we made up. A life-changing decision, as it turned out.

However, my pride had been injured, and over the next month I found myself increasingly impatient with Gerry, which I carefully hid. I even sublet a production office from *Arts in formation*, right next to his. I was in full pre-production for *The New Poverty*, which would start production on December 27. I didn't have time to break up. But I was going on vacation after the shoot was finished, and in my mind, I was planning not to see Gerry when I returned.

I decided to get a more reliable form of birth control than the cervical cap I was using. I was in my early thirties and getting fearful about infections that might limit my fertility, so I didn't want an IUD. My family doctor and I decided on the pill, and the plan was to start after my next period. Another life-changing decision.

On Christmas Eve, I was at home during the day, waiting for Gerry to call. Ange and Evelyn had gone home for Christmas. I was going to have Christmas dinner with Mary and a few other friends. Gerry and I were going to exchange presents, and he was supposed to cut my hair. The phone rang. It was

Lois, the main actor in the film, wanting another copy of the script.

From my journal:

December 24, 1986

Gerry had still not called by the time she arrived. Lois and I sat in the kitchen, knocking back rum and eggnog. I confided in her my suspicion that I was pregnant. My period was late—a rare occurrence. "Well, you're under a lot of stress with the film, it could be that," she offered.

"Maybe." I knew I was likely pregnant. December the 9th, the day the NDP elected the first MHA for St. John's East, had been the night of conception—if it had occurred. I had been working as a zone captain and hadn't expected to see Gerry. But the NDP won, so Gerry turned up at the victory party, we both got very drunk, and he came home with me after all. I know I considered putting in the cap. Why hadn't I? Too drunk?

As Lois and I discussed this, the phone rang. Gerry. Informing me that he was going out and would come by in the evening sometime. I was furious but as usual spoke in a monotone. "So you're not cutting my hair?"

"Oh, I'll do it when I come," he said. I hung up as soon as I could, and burst out to Lois. "He fucking thinks I'm going to sit around the house by myself Christmas Eve and wait for him to show up. Forget that. What an asshole!"

Within half an hour I was out of the house. The party I attended was very pleasant, tree-decorating and drink, and I stayed till 9:30. I wondered about Gerry. Had he tried to call? Christmas Eve. I relented and returned home, telling myself I could call my friend Cari in Vancouver. We chatted for half an hour. She was happy for me and my possible pregnancy.

Gerry walked in just after I had hung up. "Where were you? I've been calling all evening."

"I went out. Did you expect me to sit here all night and wait for you?"

"I didn't go. I called you back but you'd already left. I've been calling here all night. When the line was busy for so long I figured I'd take the chance and come over."

I felt mollified but also pleased that it had been his Christmas Eve and not mine that had been ruined. I got us each a rum and egg-nog, and we settled on the couch by the fire for some strained conversation. I decided to go for it, Christmas Eve or not.

"You know, Gerry, I often get the feeling that you feel you're under an obligation to see me, that you don't really want to but feel you should."

He protested. "What makes you say that? Of course I want to see you. Why else would I be here?"

"I think you feel you owe it to me, you still feel guilty over Mary, and you think you can make it up this way. I just want to say that if you'd rather not see me or you'd rather see someone else, you go ahead, and I'll do the same."

"I'm not trying to get Brownie points by being a good boy. If I didn't want to be with you, I wouldn't have come back." (Back. I hated that phrase. Come back to me. Phooey.) He continued. "Why does it have to be so complicated? I just want a simple, uncomplicated relationship."

"The only way to uncomplicate this is to stop sleeping together," I said. "That'll straighten things out very quickly."

"Well, I'm not complicated," he said. "You'll just have to take me at face value."

A white flash of anger. Icy cold. "Well, I tried that, Gerry, and you lied to me. And I haven't forgotten. So no, I don't think

I can take you at face value, because I don't trust you, and with good reason."

He went still. The Christmas tree lights looked falsely cheery. I felt very cold and hard. I wondered whether to tell him about the suspected pregnancy but decided to hold off. Why complicate things?

"I understand that," he said, "but I learned my lesson. I hope you will come to trust me in time."

"Well, only time will tell. All I know now is that I don't trust you, and without trust, there's no possibility for love, either."

Christmas Eve. How could I? But I was glad, glad to be saying it, glad to stop faking, glad to bring some congruency between my feelings and my words and behaviour. He left soon after. I opened my Christmas presents, feeling content, and went off to bed.

The Christmas Day dinner with Mary and friends was warm and comfortable. I did not blame her for any of the drama between Gerry and me, and we were still friends. She was also going to play the roommate of Lois's character in my film. Gerry and I even went to the annual Boxing Day party at Mary's. I don't know if it was tense for him, but I had fun chatting with the many guests swirling around the house. We didn't stay long, as production on my film was beginning the next day.

We started with a day of rehearsals, held at the Memorial University of Newfoundland (MUN) Extension arts space on Duckworth Street. My period had still not arrived. I told one of the actors that I might be pregnant, and by the end of the day, at least four people had asked me about it. I realized I had to tell Gerry before he heard it from someone else.

From my journal:

December 27, 1986

After rehearsal, we walked up to Dave's for an "at-home," and Gerry was there. I said to him, "I have something I need to tell you in private."

We went upstairs to a quiet room and sat on the side of the bed.

"I might be pregnant. Don't get upset, I don't know for sure. But my period's late and I have to tell you now because I made the mistake of telling someone and now the news is all over. I didn't want you to hear it from someone else first. I'm going to a doctor as soon as I can. Are you okay?"

"I'm okay. How are you?"

"I've been quite preoccupied with it, but I'm so busy with the film, I don't know. I'm fine."

He drove me home. I said, "Try not to worry about it, but if you freak out, call me."

He said, "I won't freak out, but I'll call you in any event."

On December 31, the fifth day of production, I went to Planned Parenthood on my way to set. The test confirmed I was indeed pregnant.

I was thrilled. I had always known I would like to be a mother. Now it was going to happen! That evening Gerry and I went out to The Ship, where we drank beer and shouted through the noise and smoke, then cuddled together for warmth as we made our way down to the harbour for the midnight fireworks and ship horns and back to The Hall, where we danced wildly to a local band. It had been such a fun evening, and by the time we were in bed at The Terrace, I opted for lovemaking over serious conversation. I would tell him tomorrow.

From my journal:

January 1, 1987

In the morning, before we got out of bed, I told Gerry I was definitely pregnant.

"What are you going to do?" he asked.

"Well, I'm going to keep it."

"I expected that," he said. "You told me before."

I was happy he recalled I had told him a few weeks after we started seeing each other that if I got pregnant I wouldn't have an abortion.

I asked how he felt. He said that he had been expecting the test would be positive and that he had actually told Ed about it last night. We talked, agreeing we would just have to take things as they came and see how our personal relationship worked out.

I tried to express that even if we didn't work out as a couple, that he could have access to the baby if he wanted it. He said he was a bit scared and asked how I was feeling. "You must be scared, too." I replied that yesterday afternoon I had felt weepy and anxious. But on the whole I was glad.

The shoot finished five days later. There is a Polaroid picture of Gerry and me at the wrap party, held at The Terrace. We're smiling, his hand is on my arm. He's holding a beer; I'm holding a can of Orange Crush. A picture of Pete Townsend is visible on an album cover behind us.

I phoned my mom in Ottawa. "I have some news for you. I'm happy about it, and I hope you will be, too. I'm pregnant."

"How did that happen?" she said somewhat accusingly, before throwing judgment to the wind and questioning me about my health. I was so relieved! At the end of the conversation, she said, "Well, I love you no matter what, and I'm looking forward to seeing you."

I still didn't seem to know if I wanted to be with Gerry or not. What exactly was the problem? God knows I wanted to be independent. Couldn't stand the idea of needing a man. It was hard for me to let go and relax. But reading over the journal, I'm surprised by my indecision, the fluctuating moods, in love one day, furious the next.

January 16, 1987

Gerry came to the office. I had barely seen or spoken to him all week, and I was feeling very cool toward him. I was getting ready to leave, and he said, "Let's go for supper tonight." I was instantly delighted. I said, "Wow, I'm stunned. But I'm planning to see the dance piece at The Hall tonight, it's my only chance this weekend." Then I said, "If you'll take me to supper, I'll take you to the dance thing."

We went out to The Curry House for supper. What's wrong with me? I didn't tell him I had eaten there just two days before.

We had a really nice time. I realized that it was one of the few occasions I'd been alone with him, outside of the bedroom. We need that if we're to get to know each other. We talked about the baby, I told him about my mom being so good, he said he would like to be my birthing partner. I was really pleased.

January 17, 1987

Gerry left in the early afternoon. We rarely plan to meet. He mentioned he might go to the Faustus Bidgood benefit at The Ship. I said I might too. I want to plan to see him, and at the same time I want to keep my distance. So much easier to say "might."

Why was I so unable to know what I wanted? Often, it seemed to me I had to act, even on impulse, to find out what I really felt. I relied on my mind, and my mind couldn't tell me. My mind needed my heart, but my heart needed wisdom, and that could only be gained through experience. So I blundered about.

I made an appointment to talk to Rick, my counsellor, about me and Gerry. He was a social worker with a private practice, and I had been seeing him on and off for at least a year, for what we might now call imposter syndrome. No matter my achievements, I lacked confidence in myself. I had worked on Parliament Hill for Ed Broadbent, written a master's thesis, made a well-received film, and had a Canada Council grant to make another. Still, I often struggled with feeling inadequate.

Among other causes, I blamed the Plymouth Brethren Sunday school I had attended between the ages of five and seven. The message I took away from them was that human beings would never be good enough. This had been confirmed by my Sunday school teacher. When I told her I had seen an angel, she scolded me, saying, "Who do you think you are? Angels don't appear to little girls like you."

Rick's small but comfortable office was on the floor above Planned Parenthood. I detailed the session in my journal:

January 21, 1987
Rick says, Have you had time to congratulate yourself on the film yet? I say, No, I've been really busy, I feel like I haven't had any fun in a long time, but I'm going to Ontario next week for three weeks, and I'll relax then.

We talk about the pregnancy. He makes an issue out of my statement "I want to be a single mom." He feels it has bearing on my confusion when I talk about Gerry. We talk and talk.

Rick: There are two relationships, you and Gerry as intimate lovers, and you and Gerry as parents. Don't confuse them or feel one means the other.

I tell him I can't forget about Mary, can't trust Gerry, afraid to love him. He says, talk to him about it, decide when you get more information, love takes time anyway.

Maybe it can grow if I can forgive, I think. I feel better as always after the session.

That night, Gerry and I see a play, Hadrian the 7th. *Afterwards at The Ship I feel increasingly distant. We walk home, I'm practically running in an effort not to have to talk to him. He gets in bed, I dawdle in the bathroom and get in beside him, very formal.* "Is there something on your mind?" *he asks.*

"Just the usual," *I reply. Then I got into it, saying I still bear him a fair amount of ill-will over Mary, that I am confused, that we will be parents but don't have to be lovers, that I don't know what I want but don't want to pretend. He is upset.* "Why did you take me back (Back! there it is again) if you didn't want me?" *I say because I was drawn to him and liked him.*

We talk. I question him in detail over the whole incident. He answers straightforwardly. I'm hurt, as I knew I would be, but I have to know. He lied because he panicked, he says, he was afraid he would lose me, he lied to smooth things over, he wasn't ever going to see her again, he never would have told the truth if Mary hadn't done so first.

He doesn't know, of course, that she didn't tell me the whole truth. He tripped into it, thinking she had told. Ha ha. And I pushed the table over on him, and would again, and would right this minute. I don't know if I can forgive and forget. I don't know if I could love him anyway!

I tell him the most important thing to me is not to be with anyone who causes me to doubt myself. I say I don't see much of him; I can't say whether it could grow or not. He says he's scared of me, he senses my aloofness and tries not to bug me. He wants to know what he can do to make up for it, he swears it was abnormal behaviour for him, he cares for me very much (he doesn't say he loves me). I say I'll think about it when I'm away.

We lie in exhausted silence. After a while I ask him to kiss my forehead and my eyes. Within minutes we are making love.

Is that youth? At the age of thirty-three, I had had three serious live-together relationships in my life; I wasn't totally without experience. But since I had moved to St. John's, I was more given to crushes and one-night stands—Gerry was the first relationship of any duration. And he was a nice guy, and a smart guy, and a talented guy. I loved, craved the affection and intimacy we had in bed but found it hard to be anything but distant outside. And seemingly unable to express my needs and wants. Always delaying; this isn't the time; maybe later. I would wish that I had been more honest, but it seems I really didn't know what I wanted anyway. Throw out words and see what sticks.

January 22, 1987

Thus begins a day of lazing about. It was nice. I think we didn't want to separate after the emotional conversation of the night before. We went through bookstores, for an ice cream sundae, for coffee and reading the paper, and to The Ship. At night, we went to bed, and wow—simultaneous orgasms!

We kissed and cuddled deeply for a long time. I wanted to say, I'll miss you, and I do love you—sometimes. But I always hesitate to say things like that in bed, afraid they'll seem motivated by the sex.

*We talked for a while, about pregnancy and sexual drives
and whether it was common for men to find pregnant women
sexually attractive. And eventually fell asleep. I always feel so
tender toward him in bed.*

There were other issues as well. Gerry was younger than me,
and young in the way he conducted himself. I had stayed the
night once at his house—his room was like something out of a
Fritz the Cat comic. Unwashed sheets, clothes on the floor, cold.
It all added further to the doubt side of the ledger.

January 26, 1987

*He has been at my house approximately 122 times and has yet
to wash the dishes. He makes the bed only because I told him
he couldn't come back if he didn't start making it when he was
the last one up. Now he never gets up last! He's never cooked
a meal for me, and when people are cooking in our kitchen, he
does nothing to help—doesn't even set the table. He usually
plunks himself down with a newspaper. That annoys me. How
could I live with someone like that? And why do I even consider
living with him? Just because of the baby?*

*I went to the Continental to meet Annette. She arrived just
as I did. I told her I'd begun the conversation with Gerry, but I
still didn't know what I wanted. I knew I had to tell him about
my complaints on the domestic front. She pointed out that he
probably had no idea, that such concerns were outside his frame
of reference, and that probably no woman had ever mentioned it
as a problem to him before.*

*She suggested I carefully consider the short-term benefits of
remaining in a relationship with Gerry. "What would make you
happy," she said, "washing the dishes occasionally, inviting you*

over and making his house comfortable for you to be in, going
out for a meal together once or twice a month? Tell him—it's not
much." Annette is always so sensible.

If only I had followed her advice! By now, the production office
was wrapped, I'd watched all the film we'd shot, and I was more
than ready to go on my long-planned trip to Ontario, now only
a few days away. I would see my parents, my siblings, and my
old friends. Talk everything over, maybe figure something out.
But for the moment, confusion reigned.

January 27, 1987
I just called Gerry. I'd been thinking of him fondly, thinking I'd
like to spend some time with him before I go, and thinking maybe
we could go out for supper Wednesday night. I decided I'd better
call and arrange that if I wanted it to happen, and not leave
it to chance. So I called. Instead of just saying what I wanted,
I said I'd called to see if his cold was better. We talked about that
for a while and about the big storm that had paralyzed the city
last night.

  Eventually I said something like, "I hope you're better
tomorrow, because it's one of the last chances I'll have to see
you." He went on about his plans to go to work, and maybe go
up to his mom's but go out in the evening. I felt depressed.
I said, "Well, I can't go out on Thursday." He said, "No, you've
got Sarabande practice." Then he asked when my plane was
leaving on Friday and said he could probably get the car and
take me to the airport.

  I wasn't getting what I wanted from the conversation,
because I hadn't clearly stated what that was. We continued on,
and at the end I said, somewhat pettily, "Well, am I going to see

you tomorrow or not?" He said, "Oh yeah, I'll be in the office, and I'll stay downtown tomorrow night, and I'll probably catch up with you at NIFCO.*" I hung up feeling distressed. Because I wanted something and couldn't state it.*

I imagined myself telling him I wouldn't see him before I left, refusing to go to The Ship, refusing to see him ever again or to let him see the baby. Why do I do this? Do I want him or not, or just some ideal of a relationship that can never be there with him? I might very well be better off to break up firmly with him than go on trying to mould and manipulate a relationship into something it can never be.

I have to think about Gerry when I'm away, my relationship with him, his relationship to the baby. I have to find out what he wants from our relationship, from his relationship to the baby. I have some very negative opinions of what he wants, but I haven't even asked him to express himself. Things are bad. I guess I wonder if I'm up to a relationship, let alone one that involves a baby. The whole thing makes me really anxious to go away—maybe I should stay away.

———

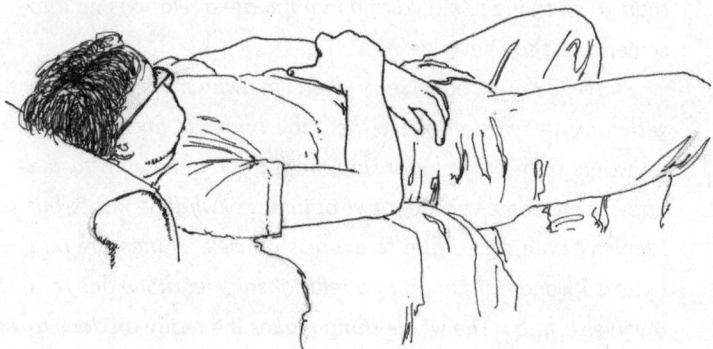

3 APRIL 88

THREE

People get cancer, and there was no reason it shouldn't happen to us. Neither Gerry nor I was bitter. We were aware of how many advantages we had compared to others in this situation. As an employee of Memorial University, Gerry experienced no break in his income but went immediately on sick leave. Because his prognosis was so dire, he was accepted for long-term disability without an inquisition. It was less money than working, but finances were never an issue for us during his illness, something I was and still am grateful for.

From Gerry's computer diary:

Thursday, May 12, 2016

- Info about pension from Michelle at HR—$49K to purchase 1 year, 8 months' service. Might be worth it.
- Chris took me to treatment /clinic for 1:30. Walked to work after for three hours of stop and chats. Nice to see Allyson and Rick, for example. Very nice. Home for International Flavours for supper.

International Flavours was a small Pakistani restaurant near Chris and Maggie's house, with a booming takeout trade. It was one of Gerry's favourites, and we often picked up their daily special to bring home both before and after his diagnosis.

As part of the bucket list, we decided to spend as much time as possible with family. Chris, Maggie, and our two young grandchildren, Jack, four, and Ursula, twenty months, lived five minutes away and ate supper with us most days, almost always prepared by Gerry. I remember Jack declaring a dance party one Saturday morning in our sunny kitchen. I joined in to the beat of "Sir Duke," by Stevie Wonder.

"Dance, Grandpa!" Jack commanded.

Gerry gamely complied, raising his hands above his head as he swayed from side to side. Did Jack's command lead to this joke?

> **NewfKarlMarx**
> @NewfKarlMarx
> There's no "I" in "Dictatorship of the Proletariat." Well there is, but you know what I mean.
> 5:05 PM - 15 May 2016

It had now been six weeks since Gerry's surgery, and we asked the oncologist if we could resume sexual activity. The answer was yes, but only if we used condoms, because chemotherapy had potentially rendered his sperm toxic. We went to the drugstore and Gerry selected the condoms to try. But we were never successful in using them, and that marked the end of our regular sex life.

Gerry was finishing and handing over his freelance website projects. He also resigned his commission as the graphic designer for the Resource Centre for the Arts. That was the hardest. He had made dozens of posters for RCA theatre productions and took delight in his creative relationship with the people at The Hall. The last poster he designed was for *Stable Home: Life with Two Horses*, directed by Lois Brown and written by Ruth Lawrence and Luke Lawrence. It had been staged just weeks before his diagnosis.

Gerry, who rarely admitted any feelings for his poster designs, suggested we get it enlarged and plaque-mounted for our new bathroom at Heart's Content.

Heart's Content, only ninety minutes from St. John's, continued to be a refuge. We drove out every weekend. Our house was across the road from the harbour, and we could watch the waves, clouds, and spectacular sunsets from our kitchen window, or venture down to the rocky beach, helping the little ones search for shells.

Using coloured chalk, Gerry drew mythic Newfoundland creatures of his own invention on the large rocks that dotted the property. Fascinated by Gerry's Lioon, a mix of loon and lion, Jack and Ursula happily engaged, creating their own designs. Working on bathroom renovations, I could hear their laughter and Gerry's encouraging words through the open back door, as I kept on staining, painting, and caulking.

Nick passed the comprehensive exams for his doctorate in Chinese history and returned to St. John's on May 19, but only for a month. He had a grant to spend the summer researching in the British Archives in London, and we did not want him to cancel.

Gerry especially did not want his health to derail Nick's progress on completing his thesis. "There's no point in changing your plans until we have something definite. Right now we're just waiting. You can take time off later, if things get bad."

We decided to plan a family vacation after Nick's research ended in August, maybe in Prince Edward Island. We'd find a big house with a beach where the immediate family could relax and spend time together. Nick's girlfriend, Caitlin, whom we had met the previous Christmas, would join us. Gerry and I would foot the bill—that's the whole point of a bucket list, spending your money on things you really want to happen. I got to work making bookings.

Nick learned the ins and outs of Gerry's routine for radiation treatments: parking as close as we could; walking to the Centre and down the stairs; check-in at Radiation reception; walking past the pleasant clinic area into the bowels of the building; sitting in the utilitarian waiting area outside the radiation chamber until the radiation therapist called Gerry in. For the half-hour or so that Gerry was inside, we usually chatted with the other people waiting.

Many of them were not from St. John's and were staying with family, friends, in hotels, or at Daffodil House, the hostel for cancer patients. We heard harrowing tales of persistent infections and repeated surgeries, emergency visits, and late-night admissions. Sometimes no one felt like talking, and we occupied ourselves with cellphones or staring at the mounted television screen. Elections were in progress in America, so there was plenty of news, most of it infuriating.

When Gerry emerged from behind the closed door, we trooped back down the long, drab corridor, into the green, pleasant clinic area, and got an appointment time for the next day's session. Then up the staircase, where we paid the parking ticket, and hopefully a short, dry walk to the car.

One day, a radiation therapist invited Nick and me to step behind the closed door. We weren't allowed to remain but stayed long enough to see lockers and change rooms and an overwhelming array of large, shiny machines, big glass windows, and staff dressed in green scrubs. It was sobering to see the white plastic-mesh mask that Gerry had to place over his face, marked with X's so they could target the radiation rays. It had screws that affixed to the bed, to keep his head in position.

A typical day for Gerry at this time can be found by looking at his Google calendar and Twitter feed. For example, on May 31 he had a blood test at 9:10 a.m., an appointment with the general practitioner oncologist at 10:40 a.m., and his twenty-sixth radiation appointment at 11:30 a.m. He also posted five photo memes about the unfolding Muskrat Falls debacle, along with twenty-one other posts on the same theme, and went to a found poetry event at The Ship in the evening.

He also found time for his alter ego. The time stamp shows he was at the Cancer Centre when he posted:

NewfKarlMarx
@NewfKarlMarx
If you're not part of the solution, you might just be non-soluble.
10:59 AM - 31 May 2016

Toward the end of his visit home, Nick dropped us off for Gerry's weekly checkup with the medical oncologist. After parking the car, he joined us in the clinic waiting area.

"I have something to tell you."

We looked at him with interest. Distractions were always welcome.

"I had a small accident with the car."

"What happened?"

"I was on hands-free, talking to Caitlin. I hit a post."

"Are you okay?"

"Yes, but there's quite a dent."

We shrugged.

We were less sanguine in the parking lot after the appointment. The bumper hung off one side of our leased Impreza, waving gently in the breeze, and there was a deep crevice across the hood. What the hell had happened?

"I opened the door to reach for the parking ticket. I had one foot on the ground for balance, but I guess I leaned so far out my other foot came off the brake and the car started to move forward." He looked down at the keys in his hand. "I put my foot back, but I hit the gas pedal instead. The car crashed into the post. And the parking arm slammed down on the hood."

"Your foot was out the door the whole time?" I said. "You could have been really hurt!"

He nodded. "Caitlin heard the whole thing. She was pretty freaked out."

"This is a total mess," Gerry fumed. "It's going to take forever to get fixed."

Gerry had always been the car guy, in charge of tune-ups and tire changes. Not being able to take charge of this situation was challenging for him. "I'll call the insurance people," I volunteered, "and Nick and I can take the car in to the dealer."

We lived in a downtown area of St. John's known as Georgestown, in between the university and the harbour and no more than ten minutes from the hospital. It's one of those colourful one-way streets that are featured in Newfoundland tourism ads. Sitting on the curb outside our burgundy row house, Nick and I used cable ties to secure the damaged bumper into position. As we tied, we marvelled that such a small event could produce so much damage.

"Anyone hurt?" said a male voice.

Looking up, we saw a middle-aged man in painter's overalls watching us from a few feet away.

I shook my head. "No, but we'll have to replace the bumper and hood."

"That's not a problem," he said. "That just takes money. A real problem is something that can't be fixed with money." He wandered off.

"Do you know that guy?" Nick asked.

"Never saw him before. You?"

"Nope."

We stared at each other in pleased disbelief. From then on, determining what was "a real problem" became part of my decision making.

Gerry's six weeks of treatment came to an end on June 6. Nick asked the radiation oncologist how much radiation Gerry had received in total. The answer was six thousand centigrays, enough that he had received his lifetime allotment. Gerry was given a schedule for decreasing his daily steroids, and we did not have to return to the Centre for six weeks. It felt like summer holidays. We celebrated by going out for both lunch and supper.

The car went in for repair, and I drove the loaner without incident. Ten days later, on June 17, Nick left for his research in London. At the airport, we took the usual selfie with the three of us at the foot of the escalator, reassuring Nick he would be the first to know if Gerry's health took a turn for the worst.

But for now, Gerry was feeling well and wanted to attend the jazz festival in Ottawa. He went every year. It was his time to visit with his father and half-brothers and to enjoy the challenging jazz music that was part of the festival's avant-garde backstage program. His festival pass for June 22 to July 3 had been purchased prior to diagnosis, and the oncologist had given him permission to fly.

This year, we decided I'd better go along too. It was only two weeks since the end of radiation treatment, and Gerry was still fatigued. We decided to stay at the Lord Elgin Hotel, right across from the main festival sites. Our room was a corner suite, with a king-sized bed and three large windows looking over Elgin Street. There was a couch, a large television, and a kitchenette. I couldn't wait to stay in a hotel, visit my family, and hear some music. I needed a break after the last few harrowing months. My family adored Gerry, and everyone was looking forward to seeing us.

It was sweltering in Ottawa, thirty degrees Celsius and humid. We paced ourselves, with no more than one family visit and one concert a day. At first, all was well. Gerry spent time with his dad, and I visited with Gail. I was relieved to see that even though I had abandoned her, she had recovered fully from her knee operation.

Over the week we saw artists Myra Melford, Sarah Neufeld, Eve Risser, Colin Stetson, and Mats Gustafsson. I was hooked. Gerry's passion for avant-garde jazz hadn't been something I shared, but I now realized we could have a wonderful time in the future. "It'd be easy to combine travel and jazz," Gerry told me as we sat in the hotel bar, sipping beer. "There are jazz festivals all over the world. In fact, there's one in Barcelona this October that I'm interested in."

Barcelona was a city we both were keen to visit. "Well, we should definitely go if you're well enough," I said. We clinked our glasses together.

On our fifth day in Ottawa, we attended a family brunch at my brother Jim's house in the Glebe. Gerry sat outside in the sun for too long, even though I implored him to put on the ball cap Jim offered. Only when his bald head was nicely red did he comply. That evening he complained of fatigue and fell asleep in our hotel room at six o'clock.

For the next two days he stayed inside, away from the heat, while I visited with friends. We went to shows in the cooler evenings. I thought Gerry was napping in the hotel room during the days but discovered later that he was also busy on Twitter. The UK had just voted for Brexit, and there was much to comment on.

> **☐☐ Gerry Porter**
> @ficklesonance
>
> Waiting for The UK to fail to invoke article 50, so we can sing
> " 🎵 Waive Britannia, Britannia waives the rules. 🎵 "
> 1:22 PM - 28 Jun 2016

A Porter family barbeque was planned for Gerry's father's house on Canada Day. Lisa and her husband, my old friend Paul Pope, arrived in Ottawa. They had decided to stay at the Lord Elgin too and came to visit in our room. They were disturbed to find that Gerry had not really eaten for two days and was nauseous and fatigued. Nonetheless, that night he came to a Porter-McGee supper held by my brother David and his wife, Anne-Marie, at their apartment, which was only a few blocks from our hotel. And he must have sent the following tweet just before we all took the bus out to his father's house in the West End.

> **☐☐ Gerry Porter**
> @ficklesonance
>
> Clicked on the CBC Feed from the War Memorial to hear a
> discussion of German armament and its ability to shoot off 500
> rounds a minute. 1/2 Something thousands of Americans can

do now with the AR-15. The entire fucking country is No Man's

Land. 2/2

11:52 AM - 1 Jul 2016

I was very concerned about him. He had been weaned off his steroids slowly and had stopped taking them entirely a few days earlier. Was this the cause? We dreaded the thought of going to an Ottawa emergency room with our complicated story. Maybe it was the excessive heat or overexertion? We were going home on July 3, and Gerry was already booked for a clinic appointment on July 7. We decided to wait for that. On our last night in Ottawa, we hosted a final family get-together in the Manx Pub, a few blocks down on Elgin. Jim, Debbie, Gail, David, Anne-Marie, Paul, and Lisa were there. Gerry had a great time, laughing and chatting, and even ate some short ribs.

The next day, Gail picked us up at our hotel at noon and drove us to the outskirts of Ottawa to see my brother Mark and his wife, Helen, who had just returned from their cottage that morning. How did we do it? Our flight home was at six o'clock. But it was important to us to see all the family members we could.

By the time we saw the doctor on July 7, Gerry had hardly eaten for six days. He was extremely fatigued, sleeping for long periods of time, and barely able to play with the grandkids. But he hadn't lost his sense of humour. In this hashtag game, a reference to alcohol is put into movie titles:

ⴹⴹ **Gerry Porter**
@ficklesonance

White Souse Down #GetAFilmDrunk

11:50 PM - 8 Jul 2016

Twelve Whiskys #GetAFilmDrunk

11:55 PM - 8 Jul 2016

How to Drain Your Flagon #GetAFilmDrunk

11:59 PM - 8 Jul 2016

Dial M for Margarita #GetAFilmDrunk

12:00 AM - 9 Jul 2016

100 Proof of Life #GetAFilmDrunk

12:08 AM - 9 Jul 2016

The Single Maltese Falcon #GetAFilmDrunk

12:25 AM - 9 Jul 2016

That same night he recounted recent events in his diary:

Friday, July 8, 2016

- Dr. M yesterday trying to make sense of this appetite loss, illness. Back on 2 mg of steroids for the time being. MRI next Thursday. Not at all doing well since midway through the trip to Ottawa.
- D and I finished *Line of Duty 3* last night. Very good. Very thrilling. Stayed up late even and watched three.
- Word this morning that Nick is safely in the UK at his flat.
- Have not felt sick today at all.
- Jack here all afternoon, mostly with Deb, but I hung out a bit too.

Many well-meaning friends offered us advice on diet and nutrition or alternative therapies as a way to beat cancer. Gerry had no time for this. He believed in science, and if it wasn't offered through a hospital or medical clinic, he wanted no part of it. There were some promising studies on immunotherapy, but the only clinical trials were in the States. Gerry did not wish to be apart from family and friends in what might be the last year of his life. He did agree to get massage therapy, though, and was astounded to discover how much he liked it.

It took a week to get the MRI and another week to get the results. By now, the steroids had increased Gerry's energy and appetite, which was good, because the Sound Symposium was on—two weeks of local, national, and international musicians and artists, presenting intriguing and unusual experiments in sound and music. I was a member of the local improv choir Vocal Explorations, and we took workshops in the day from renowned choral improvisor Christine Duncan, performing in the evening with her and our director Chris Tonelli on two occasions. Nothing is planned in an improv choir, and one night I had the opportunity to solo for a short period. I decided to reach into myself and express my feelings of grief and sadness, wailing with all my heart into the dark of the LSPU Hall.

The best part of the Sound Symposium for Gerry and me was the evening performance of *Circle of Beasts: Stockhausen's Tierkreis*, for chamber ensemble with spoken word. Our son Chris had arranged each of the twelve melodies, representing the zodiac, for piano, strings, and woodwinds, and Maggie read her poetry for each one. It was beautifully performed and well-received, and we could not have been prouder.

On July 21 we went to Leon's to buy furniture, including a bunk bed for the grandkids' room in our house, then drove to the Avalon Mall to watch a movie. At long last, it was three o'clock, time to get the MRI results at the Cancer Centre.

Again, our oncologist was direct. "The good news is there is no cancer at the surgery site."

I braced myself.

"The bad news is, there is a two-centimetre mass in the left side of your occipital lobe. It will affect your vision. There might be a spot on your spine, too. We'll order a spinal MRI to check."

Gerry and I looked at each other.

"So, more surgery?" I ventured.

"The neurosurgeon has looked at the scan. It can't be removed surgically—the risk of damage is too high."

Gerry would continue with a week of oral chemo once a month, starting immediately. An MRI every six weeks would monitor the tumour growth. He was not in physical pain, with virtually no symptoms except fatigue. How long he had left would depend on how fast the tumour grew.

Again the stagger home, the lying on the bed crying, the phone calls to loved ones. This was much worse. The first time we had hope. Now, we knew he would not be an outlier.

Gerry's computer diary that night was brief:

Thursday, July 21, 2016

- Saw *Ghostbusters* in afternoon to kill time.
- Good news / bad news regarding the MRI.
- Chinese takeaway supper with the kids.
- Chat with Nick re: MRI result.

A few days later, Tim, one of Gerry's oldest friends, came home to visit his family. Gerry and Tim had lived together for one year during university and had been fellow cartoonists and co-conspirators at *The Muse* and *Arts in formation* in the 1980s, before Tim moved to Toronto. He now had a wife and a preteen son, and they all came up to spend a night at Heart's Content. It was fun to watch Gerry and Tim competing to make each other laugh. At our house in town, we held a party in his honour, inviting their old gang from *The Muse* days. We rented glasses, bought lots of wine and beer to put in them, and Gerry made chili. His diary that night summarized the event succinctly:

Tuesday, July 26, 2016
· Very successful party for Tim. Many old hands showed up.
  Pretty beat after.

Television had always been one of the things Gerry and I did together. I had my shows, he had his shows, but the series we both wanted to watch were an enjoyable way to relax, cozying up beside each other on the couch after we had finished our work for the day. It was our "us" time. Now, this became a key coping strategy, and we watched Netflix every night we stayed at home, rapidly finishing one series and moving on to the next. Gerry's diary tells me we watched *Game of Thrones*, *The X-Files*, *The Unbreakable Kimmy Schmidt*, *The Leftovers*, *Line of Duty*, *Orange is the New Black*, *Fargo 2*, *Stranger Things*, *The Lava Field*, *Marcella*, *Heavy Water Wars*, *Bron 2*, and *Forbrydelsen* that summer.

One Sunday in early August, Gerry experienced such severe knee pain that we went to emergency. X-rays and blood work showed nothing wrong, and as the hours went by the pain lessened. We finally went home with no clue as to why this had happened.

It led to a conversation between Gerry and me on where he wanted to die. He had previously insisted he would die in hospital. He thought it would be too much fuss to die at home, citing my family's experience caring for my mom and dad. After we had been in the cold, bare examining room for several hours, listening to the distressing sounds in the halls around us, I asked if this was really the kind of atmosphere where he wanted to spend his last days. "Maybe not," he admitted.

As a result, we asked our oncologist for a referral to palliative care services. It turned out there were two ways to go. There was a Palliative Care Unit (PCU) at the Dr. L. A. Miller Centre, with a total of ten beds and three nurses. You could also get palliative care in the home through Community Services but only when a doctor had certified you were in the last twenty-eight days of life. We decided to explore both options.

We met first with the pain and symptom management team at the PCU in the Miller Centre. The Miller Centre is the main rehabilitation hospital for Newfoundland and also includes the Centre for Nursing Studies, the Caribou Memorial Veterans Pavilion, and the Recovery and Performance Laboratory, staffed by neuroscientists from Memorial University.

The Palliative Care Unit is a small wing on the third floor. The coordinator explained we could come to their clinic for visits, and they could also make house calls. A social worker was available to provide counselling to the whole family. Now that we had met with them and were on the list, we could also call the nursing desk at the PCU for advice twenty-four hours a day. We were impressed with their professionalism, and it was reassuring to have them as a resource.

I felt the knee pain might have been caused by too much alcohol. Gerry drank three to six beers every night, and I wondered if it might be interacting with his medications. I brought this up at our next clinic appointment with the general practice oncologist, a woman we had never met before. She suggested Gerry quit drinking and consider attending AA. The look Gerry gave me! On the positive side, we learned that the spinal MRI showed no tumours of any kind and that all his blood work was normal.

One sunny morning that week, I gazed out our bathroom window. The sky was exceptionally blue. The green maple trees were blowing in the steady wind, shadows flashing on the white fence, the blue hydrangeas, the golden deck. It was mesmerizing. I had a sense of deep gratitude for the beauty of life. How awful to lose this! It gave me a visceral insight into the grief Gerry must be facing, along with profound relief that I was not dying.

In August, Gail came for almost three weeks, to support me and spend time with Gerry. She slept in the grandkids' room, which was now set up with the double bed and dresser and side tables we had bought the month before. We saw plays, went to the Folk Festival, accepted dinner invitations, and spent time at Heart's Content. One evening at the Folk Festival, as I made my way to the porta-potties, I ran into a friend from NIFCO, who asked me how Gerry was doing. For the first time, I told someone outside the inner circle that he was not expected to make it.

"You guys are so brave," he said. "I don't think I could do it."

"Yes, you could," I replied. "What's the alternative? You could lie on the floor sobbing, but eventually you'd get hungry."

On August 19, we attended Ursula's second birthday party and sent well-wishes to Nick in England for his twenty-ninth. There is a delightful picture of us on Chris's balcony from that night: Jack wrapped in Gerry's arms, Ursula in Maggie's, Gail and me smiling broadly, Chris looking benign.

Gail departed on August 25 amidst many tears and hugs. We realized we hadn't taken many pictures, and Gerry obliged by doing up some photoshopped photos where he placed the three of us at the Olympics, with the *Game of Thrones* cast, and with a bare-chested Justin Trudeau. They were a big hit on my Facebook page.

It was now the end of August and time for our family retreat vacation. Nick had returned from England a week earlier, and he and Caitlin were now in PEI. The St. John's contingent flew to Halifax together, Chris next to Jack, Maggie next to Ursula, and me next to Gerry. We rented two cars and all met at our vacation rental, a gorgeous old house on the ocean near Shelburne, Nova Scotia. The weather was sunny and hot, too hot for Gerry. He did not want to be in the sun and sand, and would not come down to our private beach. Instead, he spent most of his days indoors, joining us around the campfire in the evenings. Nick and Caitlin did their best to let me have a break, and I spent as much time as I could playing with Jack and Ursula. They raced endlessly from the deck, across the field to a large rock, and back again. We made castles on the sandy beach and watched as the tide dissolved them.

And while we played outside, Gerry played inside. The following is a hashtag game putting Shakespeare references into movie titles:

ᗒᗕ **Gerry Porter**
@ficklesonance

The Twelfth Night Rises #ShakespeareSchmovies

1:54 PM - 29 Aug 2016

Hamlet The Right One In. #ShakespeareSchmovies

1:56 PM - 29 Aug 2016

Legends of the Falstaff #ShakespeareSchmovies

2:01 PM - 29 Aug 2016

Richard II: Richard Harder. #ShakespeareSchmovies

2:06 PM - 29 Aug 2016

Much Ado About The Thing. #ShakespeareSchmovies

2:08 PM - 29 Aug 2016

The Story of O. Thello. #ShakespeareSchmovies

2:11 PM - 29 Aug 2016

Love, Actually Lost. #ShakespeareSchmovies

2:18 PM - 29 Aug 2016

My younger sister Robin and her husband, Andrew, lived in the Annapolis Valley and drove down to see us for three nights, camping in their Alto trailer at The Islands Provincial Park. They visited in the house with Gerry. Robin had been wrestling with colon cancer since 2010 and had written a book on her experiences, *The Cancer Olympics*. She understood better than most of us what Gerry was going through. So many times over the years we had worried about losing Robin. Now Gerry was going to die before her. I kept myself busy taking photos as they hugged goodbye. We lost Robin in June 2024.

I thought Gerry was napping when we weren't visiting him. If I had used Twitter, I would have laughed with him about these:

Gerry Porter
@ficklesonance
I prefer to think of it as job action, not sleeping in.

9:54 AM - 29 Aug 2016

Gerry Porter
@ficklesonance
Surely it's time for the Angry Birds to move on to another stage, like Bargaining or Acceptance.

5:14 PM - 30 Aug 2016

We returned from Halifax on Labour Day. Sitting at his computer that night, Gerry called me in to the office. "John Zorn is playing at the Village Vanguard in New York City on October 9!"

"Whoa," I replied. "Our anniversary weekend."

Ever since we married in 2005, we had wanted to go to NYC for our anniversary.

"Oh man, I love John Zorn," Gerry said.

"It would be great to see him," I said.

"There's also a Paul Klee exhibition at the Metropolitan Museum of Art," Gerry said. Our bedroom was decorated with plaque-mounted posters of Klee paintings.

We looked at each other.

"You want to go?" I asked him.

"What have we got to lose? It's now or never."

Chortling with glee, Gerry immediately booked the John Zorn tickets online. I sat down at my computer and began researching plane tickets, while texting my sister Jan to ask where they had stayed on their recent New York trip. It was the Avalon Hotel, and when I looked it up online it seemed perfect for us and close enough to the venues we had in mind.

Now this was exciting! Gerry told the world about our plans:

John Zorn at the Village Vanguard! Massive Paul Klee exhibit at
the Met!

12:31 AM - 6 Sep 2016

The trip was planned for October 4 to 11, a month away. The next day, Gerry began researching hop-on, hop-off buses in New York, sending me his results via email. That night we started watching *Longmire* on Netflix, leaning into each other on the couch. Gerry must have been hopeful:

ᗒᗕ Gerry Porter
@ficklesonance

What if shit doesn't happen?

9:13 PM - 6 Sep 2016

On September 12, Gerry posted and tweeted an invitation to join him that night at the Duke of Duckworth for a celebration of his fifty-fourth birthday. I marvelled at the reach of his social media to bring out such a fine crowd on short notice. At least twenty people dropped by to see him. Many of them asked me how he was doing. I replied that we would get the results of his latest MRI in a few days, and that would let us know more.

🎧 Gerry Porter
September 13, 2016

Well, I'm incredibly grateful for all the kind birthday wishes yesterday, and a lovely evening of friends and family at the Duke last night. This little village of ours is a thing of beauty, all the more since every birthday is like some kind of crazy damn gift. Cheers to y'all.

FOUR

Pregnant and confused, the winter trip to Ottawa in February 1987 was just what I needed. My family members welcomed me, and I relaxed, visited, and napped. Everywhere I went, I was asked about the father, and I would roll out my doubts about Gerry. I thought we had no future as a couple, but should we try and live together anyway after the baby came? Of course, no one had an answer for me.

After two weeks of rest, I took a Greyhound bus to Toronto and stayed with my brother David. And here life took an unexpected turn. I went to visit Vernon, a filmmaker I had slept with on various occasions in various cities over the past two years. It had never been serious, more in the vein of the McGarrigle Sisters song "Kiss and Say Goodbye."

Vernon and I were both at a shaky time in our lives, and perhaps because of that, we connected in a way we never had before. His father had recently died, and between that and my pregnancy, we were both vulnerable and open to feeling and communicating for the first time. We talked, we shared, and our bond, which had previously been one of attraction, was transformed into one of hope and possibility. Maybe we were the solution to each other's problems?

I described what had happened in a letter to a friend:

We fell in love. I don't know why now, after all these years. But we did. I kept extending my ticket and extending my ticket until eventually I had to go home.

It was early March when I returned to St. John's, knowing I had to tell Gerry about Vernon as soon as possible, and dreading it. We had only spoken a couple of times in the month I'd been away. I called him at work, toward the end of the day. He said he'd called Toronto that morning and was told I'd already left.

"Yes, I got in late last night."

"What are you doing?"

"I've got to go to a Sarabande rehearsal tonight; we're singing at The Hall tomorrow."

"Oh, right. Well, perhaps I'll come over right now."

"Okay." This was it.

I waited. He arrived about forty minutes later—I could smell he'd gone to The Ship for a drink first.

We were alone in the house. I turned on a floor lamp in the living room, as it was getting dark. Keeping a healthy distance between us on the faded couch, we chatted about my trip, the magazine, the freelance work he'd been doing. I went to the bathroom, combed my hair, and looked at myself in the mirror. Do it. Back downstairs.

"Gerry, we have a lot of talking to do about ourselves. When do you want to do it?"

"Now."

"Okay." I sat down on the couch. "I don't know how to say this, so I'll just say it straight out. I'm very much in love with someone in Toronto, and that's why I didn't come home these past ten days."

He looked stunned. Said he didn't know what to say. I said, neither do I. "That's unusual," he replied.

He said he felt like he'd missed an opportunity. He wanted to be a father to the baby. Now he didn't know what his relationship would be.

"You're the father, and you always will be. But you never talked about living together, or taking any financial responsibility for the baby."

"I never discussed it. I thought about it. Now it's too late. I can't think about this now. Will you stay here?"

"Probably," I said. "I don't know what will happen. We'll keep talking, we'll know each other the rest of our lives, or the baby's life. We might as well start now. You can be bitter if you want."

"Oh, I don't see the point of that."

We arranged to go for supper on Saturday and talk about it then.

He left. I called Vernon at his office. Not in. I reached him at home, told him I had told Gerry.

"I just called because I wanted you to say something nice to me. I feel awful."

"It's all going to work out," Vernon said. "Don't worry, it'll be fine."

The next night I joined Sarabande for an International Women's Day event at The Hall. It was so good to see everyone. I had several close friends in Sarabande, and while I'd been away I had missed the camaraderie and the pleasure of singing.

We had an excellent performance. Could I leave Sarabande for Toronto?

That night I wrote in my journal:

March 6, 1987

We were approached by Lisa Porter, who told us how much she had liked Sarabande's performance, that we were getting tighter and tighter, and that the Witches song had sent shivers down her spine. How nice. I feel uneasy with Lisa, don't know how much she knows about Gerry and me, how much she judges. But later, as I danced wildly on the floor, she danced beside me. She put her arm around my shoulders when the song was over, and I felt warmer toward her than I have ever done. Maybe she'll be my link with the Porter family.

What kind of link I would have with the Porter family depended on where I would live, a question that was constantly on my mind. I very much wanted the baby to be born in Newfoundland. Vernon didn't feel he could make a living as a film producer in St. John's. "I could run a grocery store," he said. I had never wanted to live in Toronto and loved living in St. John's.

After much consideration, the rough plan was that I would stay in St. John's at least until the baby was born. That would give me the summer to work on my film at NIFCO. Vernon would come out for as much of the summer as he could, and we'd take childbirth classes together. He'd be present for the birth.

NIFCO had begun serious renovations during the four weeks I had been in Ontario. For the first few weeks after I returned, it was not possible for me to even go inside. But my film cans were safe in a corner, and the building was going to be great when it was finished. Could I leave NIFCO for Toronto?

Saturday came, and Gerry suggested we go for supper at Casa Grande, a Mexican restaurant on Duckworth Street. We sat at an upstairs table, where we could see the boats entering and exiting the harbour. He ordered a pitcher of margaritas. I was not drinking. Over nachos and chicken flautas, we talked for two hours. He'd just found out he had a half-brother in Ottawa—his father had a new baby in October. Wild. Gerry would have a child one year younger than his father's child. Maybe they'd be friends!

Gerry was bitter toward his father, full of blame and condescension. "You should try and deal with those feelings," I offered unhelpfully. "I've heard it's impossible to be a good parent if you have major unresolved issues about your own."

Eventually, as the pitcher of margaritas caught up with him, he began to make conversational signs of wanting to discuss "the important stuff." I looked out the window at a Coast Guard vessel docking. Finally he said, "Tell me what to do."

"About what?"

He didn't answer right away but in a few minutes said it again, and this time added, "About everything. Tell me how to live my life."

"Follow the golden rule," I said, "and then there's Evelyn's rule of 'Do what you have to do' and there's also, 'Don't do anything you don't want to do.'"

How could I be so unhelpful? I actually said that to him, poor unhappy guy.

He said, "I may seem calm, but I feel awful. I think it's terrible what's happened, really terrible. I keep thinking if only I'd said this, or if only I'd done that, things might be different. And now it's too late. That's what I can't stand—it's too late now."

"Well, it is terrible," I said. "It's an awful situation, but it's not unusual."

"It's unusual for me," Gerry said.

He continued, "After I got used to the idea of you having the baby, I really took it seriously. I did think about living together, but I thought you wanted to be on your own, and I assumed you wouldn't want to live with me. But I thought we'd work on it and see what happened, and there was some hope, and I thought we'd see after the baby was born. And I did plan on taking some financial responsibility."

"How do you see taking financial responsibility when you're going back to school?"

"The only way I can go back to school is to have some part-time and freelance work," he said. "I'll have some income. And I'm going to earn a lot in the next few months, and I'll save some of it."

"You can put it in a Pampers account," I said. "They're really expensive."

"I'm going to," he said seriously.

I asked if he had told his roommate and best friend, Ed. "No, I'm not telling anybody my personal stuff."

"Ed's going to guess," I said. "And as you know, there are other ways for people to find out than directly from you."

"Don't remind me," he said.

"At least public sympathy will be on your side."

"I don't care about that," he said. "I don't care what people think or say about my life." He went on to say he had gone out with the same woman for five years once, and they lived together for one of those years. "So I'm not a complete loss."

I knew he had not ended that relationship very well, taking up with his next girlfriend before the official breakup, but it seemed unwise to bring that up under the circumstances. He said, "I feel so young."

"You are young," I replied thoughtlessly.

His eyes narrowed. "I'm not as young as you think."

I could see the margaritas taking over, had no wish for an altercation, and sidestepped it as a discussion point. Finally he said, "Well, I won't drink any more or I'll get weepy."

He paid for the meal and we went to the Duke of Duckworth to see the Jeff Johnston Trio. They were great, and the place was packed with people I knew. Everyone was saying hello and welcoming me back. How could I leave St. John's?

My friends, as well as my roommates Ange and Evelyn, were supportive of the change in my situation. They had listened to endless hours of my doubts about Gerry, and now my declarations about Vernon and our passionate love had everyone swooning. Their delight was reassuring. I might not know where we would live, but I knew I loved Vernon, and he loved me. That certainty brought me a welcome sense of security, as I still believed that love could conquer all.

At a Sarabande rehearsal, I discussed what Mary had said when I told her about Vernon—that we were life rafts for each other at a vulnerable time in our lives. Was there something wrong with a life raft?

"Don't use words like life raft or crutch—they make a positive thing sound negative," a bandmate said. "It's the love, communication, and sharing that all people need to live, not a life raft."

Over the next few weeks, my journal entries are mostly worrying about getting the film finished, lengthy phone conversations with Vernon, and talking with Gerry. Gerry was very anxious, agitated about the whole thing, yet hadn't told a soul. I urged him to tell someone, or at least get counselling.

The NIFCO renovations were far more extensive than I had realized. I still had not been able to do any work on the film.

Vernon and I continued to write long personal letters and spend hours on the phone. He suggested if I couldn't work on the film at NIFCO, I should bring it to Toronto and find a place to work on it there. That notion both thrilled and terrified me. Vernon and I had a lot to work out. But when I thought about booking the ticket, I felt scared. I did not want to leave Newfoundland, I loved it here. I imagined throwing myself on the ground, grabbing a rock, "I'm not going, I'm not going!"

I called my friend Isabella from Sarabande, wanting to talk over my living situation. She suggested we meet at The Ship the next afternoon. Just as we were getting settled into a table, Gerry walked in and sat at the bar. Isabella and I gathered up our coats and drinks and moved to another table at the far end of the room. "The Hounds of Love" by Kate Bush was playing as we sat down.

I told her the tale, focusing on whether I should go to Toronto.

"You're asking the wrong person," she said. "If it was me, I'd be on the next plane. St. John's is too small. Look at Gerry walking in—you need more space than that."

"Should I go for maybe two weeks?"

"Go for six weeks, longer is better than shorter, you won't resolve anything in two weeks. I'm not saying you should drop your work, or saying you have nothing in your life that matters besides Vernon." She stopped to sip her beer, and continued on. "You could work something out, make a pact with yourself to work every day, even if it's just five hours. Don't let yourself slide. But I think you should go. This kind of thing doesn't happen every day. You're deep into it now. The phone can't bring anything but confusion."

Isabella made a good point, but at the moment, I had to figure out how to get along in St. John's. I complained in my journal:

March 19, 1987
I called Gerry. Talked almost half an hour with him, nice chat,
not strained. He thanked me for calling, said he'd see me on
the weekend probably.

Lois told me that Gerry stays the night at Mary's sometimes
but that Mary says they don't sleep together. I doubt that, and
if it is the case, then why have I not been invited over to Mary's
tonight along with Ed, Gerry, Lois, and a few others. Hmm?
I told Ange I felt abandoned and left out. She understood but
said that it was probably the best thing for now. I had Vernon
but Gerry had nothing, and why didn't I go for supper with her
tonight at the Continental?

Ange too made a good point. I was fooling myself to think
I could be just one of the gang, when that gang included Gerry.
I was supposed to go out with Mary the day after the party, but
when I called her, she was too hungover and instead invited me
to supper the following night.

Lois filled me in on the details of the party. They had got
incredibly drunk, everyone kissing everyone, and all of them
stayed the night. I couldn't bring myself to ask Lois but guessed
that Gerry had been with Mary. I would ask Mary when I went
for supper. I thought we would be alone, but there were other
guests, people I didn't know.

March 21, 1987
To Mary's for supper, very pleasant, but she was hiding some-
thing, and I knew she had slept with Gerry. No way to talk to
her about it, because of the company. I woke up that night at 4
a.m. and stayed awake until almost 7:30. Thinking about Mary
and Gerry mostly. Should I talk to her about it, or wait for her

*to bring it up? It bugs me that she's weird about it. I guess we're
not speaking openly anymore.*

*I talked to Ed about the situation. He says he's no help to
Gerry and can only make snarky remarks. And he doesn't know
if Gerry and Mary are sleeping together.*

The next day, Gerry called to tell me he would be able to qualify
for a student loan in September. This was good news, because
his current course had been paid for with money I had lent him
in January. We chatted, and eventually I said casually that
I might go to Toronto. I hadn't paid for the ticket yet, but it was
booked.

"It'd be nice to see you sometime," I said.

"Well, Ed and I might be having a dinner party tomorrow, and
Arts in formation will definitely have a party when the issue
comes out in two weeks."

Was he playing hard to get? "Well, I won't be going anywhere
until mid-April," I said stiffly.

Just as I was hanging up, he interjected, "I'll give you a call
sometime."

I was miffed. If he was going to be like that, I wished I had
said something about Mary, or at least about the money he
owed me. But I decided to wait and talk things over with my
counsellor before burning any bridges with Gerry.

Now I can look back and see that of course he needed to
protect himself and put some distance between us. But at the
time I wasn't overly concerned with Gerry's needs, and it didn't
take much for my indignation over what I saw as his deceit to
overcome any empathy I might have had for him.

A day later, I ran into one of the actors from my film, who
had just returned from a tour. I gave him a capsule history of

my new situation, ending by saying, "I think Gerry and Mary are seeing each other again."

"She did tell me that," he replied.

So. It was true.

March 24, 1987

It makes me want to be mean to Gerry, say something really snarky. So I can brush him away? Say you're the crumb I always thought you were, I'm not going to budge two inches to facilitate your fatherhood? Is it unfair? I mean, I dumped him and made it plain I was in love with someone else, and he can do what he likes now. He's entitled to whatever comfort he can muster, I suppose.

Still, it bugs me, rankles, that it's Mary. Did they want each other the whole time?? Is it mutual support, life rafts for each other, or is she using him even though she knows he's vulnerable? Maybe it's love. I just know I want to know what is going on and not have people hide things from me.

It's evident my feelings for Gerry were complex, to say the least. I had come of age in the free-love era, where one was supposed to be above caring about such petty things as infidelity. Most of us worked at pretending we were okay with any amount of betrayal. But as we grew older and had to reckon with the damage done, not to mention the growth of feminism and a better understanding of the patriarchy, boundaries began to be set. I still believe I would have been able to handle it if Gerry had been honest from the start. Maybe we would never have broken up!

But I also think that as time went on, I began to conflate and collapse events. The narrative I came to operate under over the next year was that Gerry had dated me while Mary was away, but upon her return he took up with her again, lying to me about it in order to keep his options open. My evidence for this position was their renewed relationship as soon as I removed myself from the triangle. In my mind, Gerry was the bad guy, I was the wronged woman, and wasn't I lucky that I had found Vernon and got out of that mess.

I booked a six-week trip to Toronto, April 12 to May 23, and began to get the film ready to travel. In those days, films were made by recording images on a sixteen-millimetre camera that was running a roll of film, and the sound was recorded separately on a portable tape recorder. In order to match an image with its sound, each take is identified using a small clapperboard called a slate. When the camera and sound recorder are both running, the camera assistant will step in front of the camera, call out the information on the slate, and then clap the two pieces together, hopefully making a clear, distinct sound. My task before leaving for Toronto was to mark the picture slates, a time-consuming job that involves finding the exact frame on the developed film where the clapperboard pieces come together, and marking each of them with an *x*, using a yellow china marker.

Luckily for me, it was now possible to work at NIFCO at night after the workers had left, and over the next two weeks I managed to get all the picture slates marked. I piled the heavy film cans in a gigantic suitcase, ready to be lugged to Toronto.

Before I left, I had a checkup with my doctor, whose office was about three blocks from NIFCO.

April 9, 1987
In terms of the baby, I feel I have really grown. Dr. C says I am
normal size for my dates, so probably no twins. I said, "I guess
all women think they are having twins at one point." He said,

"Yes, well I think all women are having twins at one point."

The most exciting thing is that the baby is moving around quite a bit. I can feel it at night, and when I am quiet, like on the bus. It feels like an air bubble, like a bloop. Usually they come in series.

I feel so blessed living in St. John's. I want to have the baby here, I want to make my film here, I want to live here. That will be the major point between Vernon and me.

Talking to Rick, my counsellor, was helpful. He was pleased about Vernon, saying I would have to give him clear permission to parent. He also said I would have to set the boundaries with Gerry and not wait for him to decide what he wanted.

Gerry knew I was leaving in a few days and asked me to lunch. He told me he had dreams about the baby, where he is filled with love and then wakes up. He picked up his fork, looking at me. "When do the birthing classes start?"

I was appalled. Surely he didn't think he would be there? I muttered something about summer. It was too much to talk about over our plates of curried beef. I did tell him that Vernon wanted me to live with him in Toronto, and that I was considering it. I didn't tell him that Vernon also wanted to talk about marriage.

On April 12 I left for six weeks in Toronto. I was now in the second trimester, and the pregnancy was becoming more obvious. Vernon occupied the top floor of a house just off the Danforth, which he shared with two other people I knew well. He and I had fun, hanging out, endless talking, playing house. I worked at the National Film Board offices in the day, now syncing the sound to the picture.

This is another exacting job. The sound tapes had been transferred to sixteen-millimetre magnetic film stock, which has frames just like the picture. This allows the sound of the clapperboard coming together to be marked and matched to the yellow *x* on the picture frame. If done correctly, the sound and the picture will be synchronized. The skill is to find the correct frame on both the picture and the sound. When I finished, it was all sent off to be edge-numbered at the National Film Board in Montreal, where I had a services grant from the women's filmmaking unit, Studio D.

Vernon was a producer on a documentary film project that would shoot in three countries in the coming fall. We agreed that he would spend the summer in St. John's with me, staying until the baby was born. After that, he would leave to manage the European wing of the documentary. When his shoot was over, I would move to Toronto.

When the six weeks were up, I returned to The Terrace in St. John's. I was still in love with Vernon but more confused. Many of the problems we faced had become clearer to me. He drank too much. He had a terrible string of broken relationships behind him and a history of affairs. Money would be a worry. It's hard to believe I didn't run screaming, but then, I was no bargain myself. Still, my journal makes for worrying reading.

June 6, 1987
I feel more negative about the whole thing than I ever have. How can this possibly work out? There's nothing in the way Vernon runs his life that attracts me, lots that confuses, depresses, and scares me. It was his willingness to see a counsellor that gave me hope things would be okay. He's stopped that now. I imagine that his drinking and self-destructive behaviour will just boomerang, and I won't want or be able to deal with it.

At the same time, I know I'm looking on the darkest, bleakest side and that my doubts are bred by the uncertainties of my own situation—baby due in three months, still unable to get into NIFCO and work on my film, worry about finances, worry about the health of the baby (a big one these days, I worry a lot about it being developmentally delayed or sick), and then the big unknown of Vernon and what is happening and will he in fact ever come this summer.

In spite of my concerns, the baby seemed fine. I could now feel frequent kicks above my belly button. Anyone seeing me would know immediately I was pregnant. I didn't like it when people patted my belly, but I did like having a baby inside me.

Since returning from Toronto, my relationship with Gerry had cooled considerably. We rarely spoke. I no longer asked anyone about his relationship with Mary, but I would occasionally see them around together. This did not please me. At the same time, it made me feel justified in my course of action. In my mind, Gerry was firmly the villain of the story.

June 8, 1987
Last night at the dance show, Gerry was there, looking grimmer and grimmer every time I see him. Later at The Ship, he came in. I don't think I spoke to him at all last night. I don't have anything to say to him, except that I'd like the $140 I lent him for school back, and that hardly seems appropriate! But why should he have it?

Later I reflected on what I want. I want him to either go away or never come out to any of the places I go to, and if he does, to never have a good time. So, that's where I'm at! Can't wait for time to pass and take care of everything.

Meanwhile, I was lonely. I longed for Vernon to come. I knew it would be tense, him and Gerry in the same small town. But I no longer cared about Gerry's feelings. I was fine to be the main villain in his story, unless he preferred Vernon for that role. We could always avoid The Ship. It was too smoky for me, anyway. Somehow we'd manage, with my friends being warm to Vernon, and Gerry's friends regarding him as an insult added to injury.

What I hadn't bargained on was the complex nature of Vernon's film production. A few weeks after I returned from Toronto, he called to say he would not be able to spend the whole summer in St. John's and would try instead for two trips. I did not take it well:

June 13, 1987

I was completely shattered. Of course, my voice began to tremble, and soon I was crying. I said that every time he called, something had changed. He said it was hard for him to give dates. I said, well, I have dates, the birthing classes start July 21, and the baby comes August 25. I said, I want to know if you're coming, so I can plan. I'd rather you didn't come and I knew about it now and could make arrangements, rather than this limbo. Don't say that, he said. And on it went, me crying, him trying to reassure; finally we agreed we would talk later that night.

I talked to Lois. She said, it's good Vernon can come at all. Me: But it's not what I wanted; it wasn't my vision. Lois: Your vision's stuck in your throat, isn't it. You're choking on your vision, aren't you? Me: Yes, this isn't a cough I've got, it's a stuck vision.

At least I had my film to work on. The renovations at NIFCO were almost completed. I participated in plastering and painting, until I realized it was probably not good for the baby. I had been assigned an editing room on the second level and instead put my energy into swabbing the Steenbeck editing machine, washing the floor, and laying down material to stop the dust from seeping back in. I put up black cloth on the windows, cleaned out a cabinet for my paperwork, and washed the cotton bags from the bin where film trims were hung during editing. The edge-numbered materials had been returned from the National Film Board in Montreal, and my first task on the film was to rewind ten rolls of sound and log the edge numbers, which are identical but incremental numbers printed in white ink along the edge at regular intervals on both the sound and the picture. When you match up the edge numbers, you know the film is in sync, which is very helpful during editing.

July finally arrived, and so did Vernon, for an eighteen-day visit. Things went well for the first while. We both were busy—he worked out of the National Film Board offices in Pleasantville, and I was now selecting takes for a rough edit. We cooked and ate at home most nights, sometimes staying in for the evening, hanging out with my roommates, and other nights wandering about Signal Hill and other St. John's tourist attractions. The Peace-A-Chord music festival was on, as well as Harbourfest. We attended childbirth classes, went to supper at my friends', and when I went to Sarabande practice, Vernon stayed home or went for a drink by himself.

Vernon and I had several arguments during his visit. They all seemed to feature the same elements: jealousy over Gerry; alcohol; and the question of whether Vernon could accept the baby as his own. Sometimes his temper frightened me. I was not used to an adult yelling at me and could only hope my roommates were not alarmed. Here is an example from my journal:

July 8, 1987

In the kitchen making tea, I could hear Vernon stomp down the stairs and out of the house, then return a few minutes later calling my name. He was in a foul temper. "I want to print this letter; I have to go to the NFB right away." "I'm making a cup of tea," I said, "and then I'll help you." "I want to do it now," he said, "you can have your tea later." "And of course, your needs come before mine," I said coldly. I made a cup of tea and carried it upstairs, feeling very hampered by Evelyn's presence in the house. There was difficulty in printing the letter because it was on the good printer and it usually takes a few tries to get new letterhead adjusted. But Vernon only had a few sheets of letterhead and became frantic when two of them were ruined. "Just do what I tell you," he shouted, "and then I can go. It's three o'clock." I said, as evenly as I could manage, "I'm not going to do another bloody thing for you if you don't get a damn site more polite. I know what time it is, I've been helping you all day, and I could have been at NIFCO." But I couldn't really have a fit because Evelyn was in the next room, and I didn't really want to break my computer, although I was tempted to throw it through the window. So, I told him to get out of my sight while I finished the letter.

There were further adventures. One Saturday we went into the LSPU Hall to look at a cartoon graffiti show. I was chagrined to find that Gerry had eight works hanging on the wall. They were funny, finely drawn, one-panel cartoons. I was surprised, because at that point I had stopped thinking of Gerry as human. Vernon, who was extremely jealous of Gerry, was outraged and left after a cursory glance. I stayed to examine them, wondering if any of that talent would be passed to the baby, who would soon be arriving.

My official due date was August 25, and I had gained twenty-five pounds. I had now moved down the hall to the biggest bedroom at The Terrace, which was quite spacious and airy. It had white wainscotting, blue-and-white flowered wallpaper, lots of room for my bed, desk, and most importantly, a dresser for baby clothes. The white crib was nestled in the large bay window that provided an impressive view of the harbour. All it needed was a baby. Speaking of which:

July 13, 1987
The baby is moving around something fierce, smashing into all parts of my body. Looks like a serpent, real David Cronenberg stuff. They Came from the Inside.

A night or two before Vernon was to return to Toronto, we had a barbeque party at The Terrace.

July 23, 1987
Someone told a story that mentioned Gerry's name. Sure enough, Vernon immediately went upstairs, came down a bit later, and went out and bought beer. I went to The Ship after Sarabande practice, and Vernon came in. I motioned him to our table but found he was drunk. In fact, he was completely drunk, almost falling on my friends. I was humiliated and angry. We left, him rolling and falling against me on the way up the hill. I stayed outside while he went in the house.
I went in after almost an hour, to find Vernon lying on the floor in my room, fully clothed and snoring loudly. I just left him there. Sometime during the night, he got up and came to bed. In the morning we had words. I said it wasn't working

out, he wanted to know if it was over, I said I had to go for the
Sarabande performance. He missed most of the performance.
Afterwards we talked, sitting on an outside bench. We decided
it wasn't over yet.

A few days later, Vernon returned to Toronto for two weeks. It was the third week of July, and I was due in a month. I didn't discount the possibility that things would not work out with him. I wanted passion and love but not necessarily the amount of drama that accompanied Vernon. But it seemed reasonable to wait until the baby was born and see how Vernon reacted. He could be patient and reassuring, and when we cuddled, all was right with the world. Plus, he was helpful with my film, watching it on his own and making notes and useful suggestions. I still felt positive about him, in love and loved.

My roommates were not concerned about Vernon and his behaviour. Living arrangements were fluid in our communal household, and none of us planned to live together forever. I knew neither of them really warmed to him, though he seemed to get on well with Ange's current boyfriend. But they knew Vernon would not be at The Terrace on a permanent basis, and as Ange said, "Why did I need to like your lover anyway?"

I also talked to my counsellor, Rick. He talked about "areas of responsibility," that Vernon had to deal with his problems, and I with mine. Not to tell people how they should be but rather decide for yourself what your boundaries are. He also said not to get fooled by the potential of a situation but rather accept and deal with the reality. He thought I was wise to be asking these questions about Vernon and me.

Vernon came back on August 3. I was happy.

August 10, 1987
I don't worry too much about how he will react to the baby.
He's been excellent around the classes and the doctor's
appointments and seems very interested in my health. We
had to get baby stuff on the weekend, and he was enthusiastic
about refurbishing a change table we bought, and when we
sorted through the pile of baby clothes, he was quite taken with
several of the cute little outfits. We'll see what happens around
the birth and first weeks of life.

On the morning of August 17, I was in the editing room at NIFCO when my water broke. Vernon and I taxied to the maternity hospital, and I was swabbed for amniotic fluid. Swabs are supposed to change to blue immediately in the presence of amniotic fluid, and my swab did not. I was sent home. I couldn't get a clear explanation as to how I would know when it was amniotic fluid, since I couldn't conceive of being wetter than I was.

The next night, after birthing class, I told the instructor that I had continued to drain fluid all day.

"Go up and get checked again," she urged. Again, the swab was negative. As we sat in the examining room, discussing what might be going on, one of the nurses pointed at the tray—look! The swab was slowly changing to blue. It must be defective, someone said. This set off alarms. What if my first swab had also been faulty? The baby could be in danger of infection. I was admitted immediately. If labour did not begin on its own overnight, I would be induced the next morning.

Despite a few weak contractions, at eleven a.m. on August 19, 1987, I was started on an oxytocin drip.

The labour was very painful, as my cervix went from no dilation to full dilation in a matter of hours. Vernon was great, taking photographs, holding my hand, his face right over mine whenever I would open my eyes. I hadn't wanted to have painkillers or an epidural, but the force of the contractions quickly changed my mind. I accepted Demerol.

In between contractions I was woozy. I wanted to know what stage of labour I was in, to get some idea of how much longer it would go on. "Do you think the baby will be born today?" I asked, and the nurses laughed and assured me it certainly would.

It was time to push. Everyone was yelling, push, push! "I *am* pushing!" I yelled back.

Suddenly the fetal monitor began beeping, indicating the baby was in distress. Just like on television, amidst cries of "We've got to get this baby out!" I was transferred to a stretcher and rushed down the hall to the operating room, ceiling lights flashing past my eyes. "Don't push, don't push!"

The baby was too far down the birth canal for a Caesarean, so an episiotomy was performed and forceps inserted. Then it was "Push, push, push that baby out! You'll have the baby on the next push!" I was pushing for all I was worth, making an unholy racket. Push, push, push, screaming, then the head, an immediate sense of relief, then, "Your baby is born." It was two o'clock in the afternoon.

I was so certain I was having a girl, I was confused when they told me I had a son. Was my baby actually born? It took me a minute to grasp that my baby *was* a boy. A rush of events around the baby, the blue cord which apparently had been wrapped around his neck twice, a memory of his body being placed across my chest and looking at his beautiful, tiny face.

The placenta was not in good shape, seeming to confirm that my water really had broken earlier. My doctor said they wanted to be very careful with the baby, because the chance of infection was high. He would be checked out in the neonatal nursery. Then he was gone, and I was wheeled into the recovery room.

———

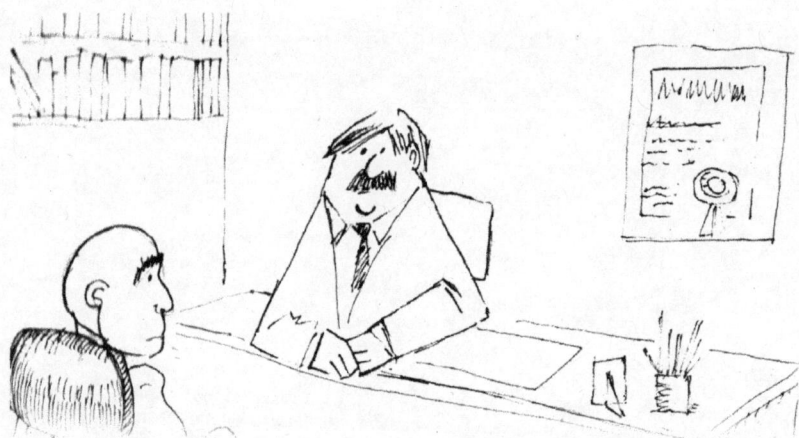

"I'm sorry. I'm an ontologist. I can't treat your cancer, but I can prove you exist."

@FICKLESONANCE

FIVE

On September 15, 2016, Gerry and I were sitting in the Cancer Centre, waiting for the MRI results.

The occipital tumour had doubled in size. If it kept growing at this rate, Gerry would have two months to live.

"Why can't the tumour just be there?" I pleaded to the oncologist. "Why does it have to kill him?"

The answer was that the tumour would grow until it pressed so heavily on his brain stem that life functions, such as breathing and heart pumping, would be cut off. There was no arguing with that.

Gerry's monthly chemotherapy would be discontinued. It wasn't making a difference.

"I don't think your cancer is chemo-sensitive," said the medical oncologist.

The original site in the temporal lobe was still cancer-free, indicating that the cancer was responsive to radiation. The radiation oncologist suggested a five-day secondary radiation treatment, targeted on the occipital lobe. It might slow the growth and give Gerry more time.

Again, the staggering, the crying, the phone calls. It was unbelievable to both of us that he would die, and sooner rather than later.

"I don't want to waste time on television shows that might not be good," Gerry said. "From now on I just want to watch *The Wire* and *Buffy the Vampire Slayer*. Maybe I can get them all in."

Gerry's diary entry that evening:

Thursday, Sept. 15, 2016

· Lunch at International Flavours with the b'ys from work: Rick, Benj, Adrian, Steve, and Jamie.
· In receipt of the bad news from Dr. L. Fucked-up day all around. We did speak to Nick and Chris, but that's all.
· Started *The Wire* rewatch. Not much of a supper.
· McNulty: I am fucked. Fucked is me.
· Can't write anything today. Can barely see.

Gerry's diminishing eyesight would soon take centre stage, but the next day we had a home visit from the social worker with the Community Services palliative care team. We sat at the kitchen table with steaming mugs of tea. He prompted us with timely questions such as: Is your funeral arranged? Burial or cremation? Do you have a do-not-resuscitate order in the home? Is the obituary written? Is a doctor lined up to pronounce on death should it occur at home? I wrote these questions down in The Gerry Book, calling it "The Sad List."

Gerry's diary that night was as emotional as it got:

Friday, Sept. 16, 2016

· Spoke to Dad today. Spoke to Lisa earlier. Not an easy day at all. Brutal, actually.

· May have solved some of the stupid wireless problems. Maybe.

· Two more eps of *The Wire* season 1.

My youngest sister, Jan, a librarian, and her husband, Paul, a visual artist, were flying in from Rockwood, Ontario, to see Gerry. They had booked the tickets in July, back in the halcyon days when we still had hope he could live for two, or even five years. They would arrive the next Friday and spend the weekend with us. That gave me a few days to start on The Sad List.

We began with our family doctor. To my surprise, she would not take responsibility for the DNR order or for pronouncing Gerry's death should it occur in our home, saying, "You already have people for that." I suppose she meant palliative care. My feelings were hurt. She had been looking after us for twenty-five years.

Well, could I get sleeping pills for myself? Since the two-month timeline had been introduced, I was finding it increasingly difficult to fall asleep and often woke up at four a.m. I would lie awake next to the slumbering Gerry, adrenalin coursing through my body, and only fall asleep when the sky lightened.

Gerry's vision continued to deteriorate. It was becoming difficult for him to work on his computer and even to cook. The protocol for getting services from the Canadian National Institute for the Blind (CNIB) was to get a referral from your optometrist, after which it could take up to six weeks to get an appointment. Clearly that time frame was not going to work for Gerry. I had become shameless about getting to the front of the line by plainly stating why we needed special treatment. We got an appointment to meet with the intake officer at the CNIB two weeks later, on September 30.

By now I was snatching at time to get everything ready for Jan and Paul's visit the next day. Our Subaru hatchback was covered in dust and dirt. I vacuumed the inside, but a trip to the car wash was also needed. This had always been Gerry's job, and I was not keen to have him as an on-board critic. Nonetheless, I suggested we stop at the car wash near the hospital on our way to the first of the new radiation appointments.

Things move quickly once you're in the car wash. There was a sign with directions, instructing me to punch in our entry code, put the car in neutral, and turn off the engine. There were some lines of text I didn't have time to read because suddenly the wide glass doors rolled up, the car magically moved forward on its own, and we were blasted with jets of water. Then soap was slopped over the windows, and I couldn't see. We were jerked forward for more blasts of water and suddenly we were propelling toward the drying area. There was another sign with more directions I missed, and suddenly the car stopped half-in and half-out of the rolled-up glass exit door. Warm air blew ineffectually on the glistening burgundy surface.

"You went too far forward," Gerry said.

I made a split-second decision to back up and prove I could do it right. As I reversed, the quickly descending glass door smashed into the back window. The car shook. Zillions of shatter lines appeared, looking absurdly beautiful in the sun. Then the entire window fell into the freshly vacuumed hatch.

There was a moment of silence as we both pondered this turn of events. I looked at my watch.

"We've got to go! It's almost time for the appointment."

I sped off. It was a nice day, and the breeze from the back was not unpleasant. Gerry remained silent, no doubt torn between moral support and moral outrage. I felt strangely light-hearted. This was not a real problem—it could easily be fixed with money.

That night Gerry decided it was time to notify key people in his life about his diagnosis. He began with an email to his poker buddies.

Thursday, Sept. 22, 2016

Poker lads!

An email to bring y'all up to speed on my health, mainly because news is slipping out, and it's not good.

Basically: a new and big-ass tumour has developed on the opposite side of my brain, in the occipital lobe. That's causing the vision problems I mentioned at the last card game. Anyway, it's a beast and not at all unexpected, because that's what this illness does. They started a secondary short course of radiation today with hopes of shrinking or slowing its growth. But the best outcome here adds weeks, not months, to the prognosis. Sucks, I know, but we're doing okay, having been prepared for this since May. So fuck it. We keep going on until we don't. I can still play cards (probably poorly), and to that end I think Ed will be in touch soon about a game maybe a week from Friday.

Thanks to Speedy Glass, the car window was fixed by the time Jan and Paul arrived at eleven o'clock the next morning. Gerry and I picked them up at the airport, and I placed their luggage in the once again pristine hatch. "So, first we have to go to the Cancer Centre for Gerry's radiation treatment," I said. "It won't take very long."

"Yeah, we've planned a tour of the top cancer sites in St. John's," said Gerry.

"Actually, I'm kind of interested," said Jan.

Gerry's second radiation treatment was in a room new to me, and it turned out I knew the radiation therapist. I introduced her to Jan and Paul before she and Gerry disappeared behind the very thick door. The three of us looked at each other and sat down to wait on the comfortable yellow couch. "So, how are the kids doing?" I asked, referring to my nephews Palmer and Kadin, both still living at home. I was all caught up on their exploits by the time Gerry was ready to go.

We went home for lunch, and I showed Jan and Paul to their room. "Do you think you guys could help me put the upper bunk in place before you go?" I asked. "We bought it in July, but after getting the main bed assembled and the dresser in place, there just hasn't been time. It's set up in the next room."

"Sure," said Paul. "Happy to be useful!"

But more important things first. Neither Jan nor Paul had met Maggie, Jack, or Ursula before, and we all spent the afternoon at our house, playing games with the grandkids. Gerry went for a nap while I demonstrated "obstacle course," a game Jack and I had perfected that involved jumping from couch to piano bench to couch, while gathering small stuffed animals along the way.

That night we dined on International Flavours and chatted in the living room. We told them about The Sad List. They told us about the new building Paul had bought in Alton, a small town near their house. "It was a church, then the Alton town hall," he said, "I'm in the middle of renovations."

"So will it be an art gallery?" Gerry asked.

"Yes, a place to sell my art but also to hold weddings, receptions, concerts, even film screenings."

"You can google it," said Jan, "Paul Morin Studios."

The next day was Saturday, and as there were no radiation treatments on weekends, we decided on an overnight trip to Heart's Content, leaving around one o'clock. On the way, we listened to a playlist Paul had put together for Gerry. It was warm and sunny when we arrived, and Gerry had enough energy to walk to the nearby government wharf to count the fishing boats but not enough to continue on to the lighthouse. Instead, we drove there, admiring the ocean and the clouds. We spent the evening drinking red wine at the kitchen table.

"You know, we should do something special tomorrow night," I said.

Gerry poured a little more wine into Paul's glass. "That's a good idea," he said, "but it's Sunday."

"What about going to The Reluctant Chef for the tasting menu?"

"What's a tasting menu?" said Jan.

"Oh, it's really cool. The chef decides what you're going to eat," said Gerry. "You let them know if you have any allergies or strong dislikes, and they bring you out small plates. It's usually five courses, including dessert."

"So you all eat the same thing?" said Jan.

We nodded.

"And we could do a wine pairing with it," I said. "The sommelier decides what to serve with each course, and they come out and tell you what it is and why they picked it for that dish."

"Sounds fun," said Paul, raising his glass.

"I'll call tomorrow morning and see if we can get a reservation," I said.

Unfortunately, that night, Gerry had another crushing bout of knee pain at three a.m. I got up to run him a hot bath but was so tired I went back to bed once he was in the tub, where he spent the rest of the night.

In the morning Gerry was again pain-free. I called The Reluctant Chef and reserved a table. We drove into town with enough time to get spiffed up and down to the restaurant, on Duckworth Street, not far from The Ship.

We were seated on the second floor, at a round table with a royal blue tablecloth, red cloth napkins, and an eclectic mix of china place settings, which gave the atmosphere a nice mix of elegant and funky. Our server for the evening was the daughter of a friend of ours, and it was lovely to introduce her to our family. And then the meal began. Each course she brought out was like opening a Christmas present. What have we here?

Looking back, I can't recall the food. But the photographs on my phone reveal an appetizer of red tuna tartare on a large wonton, a course of soup that might be pumpkin or squash, garnished with crispy shallots, and a main course of duck breast with savoury braised navy beans, orange marmalade, and balsamic onions. What I do recall is the laughter, the pleasure of being together, and our delight as each new dish was unveiled, each new glass tasted. Thank goodness we had chosen the three-ounce wine pairing, because after five glasses we were quite tipsy. On the way out, Jan said to me, "I didn't realize Gerry's eyesight was so bad. I just redirected him from the ladies' room."

The next morning, Jan and I assisted Paul in moving furniture around the bedroom, then left him to assemble the bunk bed on his own. The bottom was a double, and the single top bunk very close to the low ceiling. But I knew Jack and Ursula would love climbing the ladder. I then took Gerry to radiation.

Their plane was leaving at five o'clock, and before we drove them to the airport, they gifted Gerry with a marijuana cigarette. "It could help with pain and probably anxiety, too,"

Paul said. Inside the terminal, we said goodbye at the foot of the escalator leading to security. Gerry hugged them, first Paul, then Jan. "Thanks for coming, guys," he said.

"It was a blast," Paul replied. "Thank you!" They waved at us as they were transported up the escalator.

We held hands on the way to the car. "Let's watch *Buffy*," Gerry said. I nodded.

By the time the last radiation session was completed on Wednesday, September 28, Gerry was beginning to find himself off-balance upon standing. "How are you feeling about New York?" I asked. The trip was still five days away. He sighed and put his phone down.

"I don't think I can do it," he admitted. "I don't think I'd be able to handle the waiting at security and customs. And I can't see well enough to look at anything in an art gallery."

The next day, I cancelled our plane tickets and hotel reservations, and Gerry cancelled the Village Vanguard. That evening he tweeted:

ᴖᴖ **Gerry Porter**
@ficklesonance

Hottest trend for next quarter expected to be the fetal position.

9:49 PM - 29 Sep 2016

We were sad, but we were not devastated. Our skill in ascertaining what was a real problem, one that no amount of money could solve, had been developing. Cancelling New York did not rate. Our real problem, the tumour pressing down on Gerry's brain stem, was becoming more and more evident, and dealing with it on a daily basis didn't leave much time for disappointment.

For example, the appointment at the CNIB the next day was very successful. Gerry was going to be a short-term client, but they still had plenty of services to offer. We came home with task lights and a variety of magnifying glasses. Grandson Jack favoured the classic Sherlock Holmes type, using it to play insect detective in the covered sandbox Gerry had built in our backyard. Carpenter beetles loved the sand too, and when Gerry opened the hinged lid, Jack squealed in excitement at the small, grey bodies fleeing from the sunlight.

That night, Gerry elected to play cards instead of attending the Jerry Seinfeld show we had tickets for. I went with Susan Shiner (it was very funny). I found out the following year, when I read his diary, that Gerry had got lost while walking to the game, even though it was only three blocks from our house. He'd had to call his friend Johnny to leave the game and come and get him.

How did Gerry react to this? His online diary for that day reads as if it was a small thing:

Friday, September 30, 2016

· CNIB first thing, then breakfast at Jumping Bean.
· Very successful poker game, except for getting lost at the beginning.

Late that night he tweeted:

◯◯ Gerry Porter
@ficklesonance

The best thing about spending an evening with your best mates is they don't GAF.

1:55 AM - Oct 1, 2016

The next evening, October 1, we attended a dinner party with some of Gerry's oldest friends, including two people who had been at the poker game the night before. The first part of the evening involved walking through a wooded path to a small pond, where we gathered around a fire, munching appetizers. I was concerned about Gerry's safety near a pond and a fire. To preserve his dignity, I did not physically help him but let his buddies know how poor his vision was. "Oh, we know all about it," they said. "We're watching out for him."

What do I think about it now? I'm glad for Gerry that he was able to cope with this significant loss of independence with the collusion of his friends, and with his signature humour:

ᗡᗡ **Gerry Porter**
@ficklesonance
I tried to board the emotional roller coaster, but I think I ended up on the emotional clown car instead.
2:14 AM - 2 Oct 2016

I'm also glad we had the CNIB, which continued to provide services. That week, the IT specialist came to our home and, sitting with Gerry at his computer, installed accessibility software. Gerry's cellphone was modified with large font. The low-vision specialist showed him tips for cooking safely and gave me lessons on how to assist Gerry when walking outside.

Gerry decided to go public with his worsening vision:

ᗡᗡ **Gerry Porter**
@ficklesonance
BTW if you see me IRL and I seem weird or distant it's because my vision has declined a lot lately because of tumour mischief. It ain't you.
9:05 PM - 4 Oct 2016

On The Sad List front, we got a signed do-not-resuscitate order from the pain and symptom management team at the Miller Centre. That visit gave me a few new tasks: getting a disability parking permit and ordering medical marijuana to help relieve pain and anxiety. Gerry felt he had benefitted from the marijuana gifted by my brother-in-law and wanted to add it to his daily regime.

October 8 came and our wedding anniversary was celebrated at Raymond's, a high-end restaurant we had never been able to afford. Courtesy of a gift from my aunt, we booked a table. We weren't in New York, but we dressed up, Gerry in a suit and tie and me in pearls and an autumn dress of burnt orange. I also wore the earrings I had worn at our wedding eleven years earlier. The restaurant was in a heritage building, and the room was spacious, the atmosphere relaxed, even quiet, despite every table being occupied.

We again chose the five-course tasting menu with wine pairing. The blends of flavours in each course were exquisite and the plating so imaginative, it was hard for Gerry to separate the food from the decorations, especially the first course of caplin with salsa verde, seared whelk, and a fresh BC oyster served on a cross-cut section of tree trunk. By the time we were sipping the glass of wine paired with our fourth course, we could no longer discern if it was oaky, flinty, or earthy, and we didn't care. Before we left, the pastry chef gifted us with a plate of bite-sized sweet biscuits, carefully arranged alongside two mystery objects wrapped in translucent paper. Written across the plate in a flowing script of dark, thick chocolate sauce were the words Happy Anniversary. We look pleased, and perhaps slightly tipsy, in the picture taken by our server.

Very late that night, Gerry posted on Twitter:

🤓 **Gerry Porter**

@ficklesonance

Raymond's genius or blindness I'm not sure, but I ate stuff
tonight I never would have touched before, like whole caplin
and oysters.

3:09 AM - 9 Oct 2016

The next day we recovered from our excesses in time to have
a Thanksgiving turkey dinner with the family at Chris and
Maggie's. On Monday, returning to The Sad List, I texted my
sister Jan.

October 10, 2016, 8:34 p.m.

–Would you consider making an urn for Gerry?

–Of course, dearest. You'd need to give me some
direction. Do you want the same box as I used
for Mom's?

–I will ask him. This is his request—he really likes the idea of
an urn made by family. Sniff.

–Okay, anything for Ger. If he could think about what kind
of design he'd like, that would be a great place to start.

–He says he admires your aesthetic and would like a nod to his
Scottish heritage through some Celtic lettering and imagery.

In peak Sad List mode, Gerry and I visited Carnell's Funeral
Home one afternoon in mid-October. An assistant funeral
director ushered us into a bright glass-walled room, where we
sat at one end of a large wooden table. He showed us binders of

caskets and flower arrangements, and in the end we purchased a package that included a cremation and three visitation sessions, scribbling our signatures on the paperwork. We high-fived when we exited their building. We have the cremation and wake paid for! Yay us! Oh.

Gerry was a militant atheist, and I am a Buddhist. There was no way he was having a church funeral. Instead, we decided on a memorial gathering, an affair that would be a chance for remembrances, music, food, and drink. A week after visiting the funeral home, I met with Kelly, an owner of Rocket Bakery and its event space, The Rocket Room, located on Water Street. I instantly liked her, and she was very open to holding a memorial service instead of their usual wedding and anniversary parties. I obviously couldn't make a firm booking, but I came away with the price list and a rough idea of how such an event might quickly come together.

There are no more journal entries from Gerry after October 12, but he continued to post on Facebook and Twitter. Invitations to socialize over supper were pouring in, as were offers to drop off meals. We accepted the invitations but preferred to do our own cooking at home as long as possible.

On a Sunday afternoon in mid-October, a friend of ours from Gerry's work (where I had also worked before retirement) held a potluck party for Gerry at her home in Mount Pearl. Thirty or so colleagues, past and present, turned up. Several took me aside to tell me of the kind things Gerry had said or done for them over the thirty years he worked at the university, from assistance during a personal crisis to making a CD for their child. The next day, many pictures were posted on Facebook. I look grim in most of them. Gerry, however, with his full red cheeks and big belly (courtesy of the steroids) looked healthier than he had most of his life, when he was almost gaunt from his heavy smoking.

Nick arrived on October 17, intending to stay until the end. From now on we would always have company.

"I'm kind of sad," I told Gerry. "I'm going to miss being alone with you."

But I was also glad to have help and someone to confer with. It was getting harder to manage the house and food and all the appointments by myself, and Gerry was now relying on a cane for support.

Gerry's father flew in the same night Nick arrived, intending to stay with Lisa for a week. David, one of their three half-brothers, came for a few nights as well. We had dinners at Lisa's, dinners at The Ship, dinners at our house. One afternoon, Gerry and his dad stretched out on our bed upstairs, watching science shows on Netflix. They kept calling out for help with the remote control.

Jack was downstairs, playing games on the iPad, and since he didn't read, frequently needed assistance. I was making supper, and Nick was tasked with running up and down the stairs, patiently tending to the young and the old.

"Looking after people these days seems to be mostly a matter of tech support," he commented.

That same night at our supper table, Gerry's dad abruptly stopped speaking in mid-sentence, put his head in his hands, and began sobbing. I was busy at the stove, and Gerry awkwardly patted his dad's shoulder, shooting me helpless glances. I thought it was probably good for him to cry. It was a sad situation, to be in your eighties and know your son was going to die before you.

His dad was happier two days later when Gerry's first cousins on his mother's side had an afternoon potluck get-together in Blackhead, near Cape Spear. Gerry's mother had been born in

Blackhead, and I liked to refer to it as their ancestral homeland. It was the first time in thirty-five years that Gerry's dad had seen many of the guests. Apart from the underlying sadness at the reason for the gathering, it was a fun family event, with two-year-old Ursula and five-year-old Jack rushing about examining decorations for Halloween and the rest of us laughing, talking, and eating. Perhaps this was behind Gerry's tweet:

NewfKarlMarx
@NewfKarlMarx

Christ, the dustbin of history is overflowing onto the floor here.

5:46 PM - 22 Oct 2016

October is also when the annual St. John's International Women's Film Festival is held. I had bought tickets for Nick, Gerry, and me to see the closing night screening of the St. John's premiere of *Maudie*, about Nova Scotia folk artist Maude Lewis, on October 23. It was produced by our friend Mary Sexton, and we all wanted to see it. Unfortunately, during supper at our place that night, Ursula fell off her chair, hitting her head on the stove. She cried so long and hard her parents decided to take her to the children's hospital. Nick volunteered to look after Jack, and Gerry and I guiltily went off to the film screening at our local Cineplex. Nick would have other chances to see it, but this was probably Gerry's last opportunity. We arrived late and had to sit in the front row, which turned out to be the best place for Gerry. The film, which is a reluctant love story, ends with a hospital deathbed scene. We cried, of course, and escaped through the crowds afterwards as quickly as we could. (Ursula was fine, by the way.)

Nick, Chris, and I had been discussing some way to commemorate Gerry. Instead of a park bench with a plaque, or a theatre seat with Gerry's name on it, we wanted to set up a grant or award. Maybe something to do with posters or graphic art? Gerry approved the idea but wanted the grant to be for the kind of improv music he loved. We invited our friend Mack Furlong from the Sound Symposium to come to our house on October 24. Between us all we hammered out the details.

It was to be called The Gerry Porter Award for Creative Improvised Music, valued at one thousand dollars and given every two years at the Sound Symposium to "an individual, group, or organization based in Newfoundland and Labrador that produces or supports challenging music created by the will and spirit of the practitioner, known as creative improvised music."

I made inquiries with the Community Foundation of New-foundland and Labrador. It would take fourteen thousand dollars to endow the award. The plan was to ask for donations at the memorial service and use Gerry's life insurance to make up the difference.

We also decided to use his life insurance to buy a good violin for Maggie and a good saxophone for Chris. The budget was twenty thousand dollars for the two of them. Gerry was deeply pleased to make this offer. Because we were nothing if not fair, Nick would be given ten thousand dollars to do with as he wished.

I got word that our medical marijuana request had been approved. Neither Gerry nor I were dope smokers, and it was confusing to figure out how to fill his prescription. Cannabis was not legalized in Canada until 2018, and I had to pick a provider from a dozen or so licensed companies set up across the country, which meant looking at a dozen or so web sites. The range of product was bewildering. Did we want high, medium, or low

THC? How about high, medium, or low CBD? What strain did we favour, Indica or Sativa? Perhaps we would prefer to ingest oil instead of smoking? Of course, Gerry made a joke about it:

ᴗᴗ **Gerry Porter**
@ficklesonance
Sorting through the medical marijuana situation in Canada is making me consider starting a medical scruncheons, gravy, and dressing service.
6:23 PM - 25 Oct 2016

I finally chose a mix of CBD and THC, all medium, one in oil and one in marijuana. The product arrived quickly, and Gerry was soon looking forward to his nightly bedtime vaping. I tried to join in but found the effects too unpredictable. I was just as likely to stay up all night as fall asleep. I gave up, leaving it to Gerry, and sometimes Nick.

On October 26, just before bed, Gerry left the living room to put his mug away in the kitchen. Crash! We sprinted in, to find him on the floor. "I slipped," Gerry said. Whatever had happened, he banged his head hard enough to draw blood. Nick and I exchanged glances. From now on, someone would always have to be near him.

It had now been four weeks since the end of the secondary radiation, and Gerry went for an MRI to see if it had helped slow the growth. That night, our friends Gerry Rogers and Peg Norman had invited us for dinner, along with Ed and his wife, Frances, and Paul and Lisa. Everyone was close enough to us to know our situation, and the dinner table conversation was about the pros and cons of venues for the memorial service. Gerry Rogers told us about a friend who had attended his own wake, held at his house. Paul said hesitantly, "Have you thought of having it while you're still around?" There was instant enthusiasm for this notion. A celebration of Gerry's life while he was still living it!

"We could call it Gerrypalooza," I said.

A day later, Gerry said, "Remember what we talked about at dinner? I like that idea. Let's do it."

The chosen date was Friday, November 25. Now we were planning a big party, very different from planning a memorial service. Nick and I went down to The Rocket Room to discuss details with Kelly, the owner. "A pre-mortem party," she said. "What a great idea!" The plan was to display Gerry's artwork and posters in a slide show, hang some of his mounted work on the walls, have a guest book, speeches, and music. It would be wonderful. We had three weeks to get ready.

Life wasn't all about cancer—there was still time for fun with the family. While Gerry attended his friend Benjy's birthday party, Nick and I took Jack and Ursula to an extravagant *Sesame Street* show at Mile One Stadium. They were transfixed by the singing and dancing giant Muppets. It was good to have an evening of sweetness. Then came Halloween. Jack was Raphael, the red Ninja turtle, and Ursula was Batman. Nick and I tended the door. Gerry stayed upstairs for most of it, amusing himself and others on Twitter:

ᗒᗕ **Gerry Porterr**
   @ficklesonance

Oh cool. Newfoundland just came to the door dressed as a
boondoggle. Some cute.

6:38 PM - 31 Oct 2016

ᗒᗕ **Gerry Porter**
   @ficklesonance

Future Halloween costume idea: drag a small house on a wagon
behind you and call it resettlement.

6:41 PM - 31 Oct 2016

👓 **Gerry Porter**

@ficklesonance

Shelled out, b'y. Nothing left but an abiding love of
Newfoundland and Labrador.

8:03 PM - 31 Oct 2016

When he wasn't playing on Twitter or napping, Gerry had been
creating a music playlist called "Music for a Possible Event."
Now that the event was Gerrypalooza, he had a concrete dead-
line to work toward. Nick was helping to either close Gerry's
websites, or transition them to the appropriate people. In
Ontario, Jan was carving the urn.

November 2, 2016, 12:51 p.m.

– Hello there! More questions: Do you want Gerry's name
on the urn? What is his full name? Is there a saying you
would like added?

– He says WTF, but don't use that.

😂😂😂

– So far: Gerald Cameron Porter. He says "Caution – contents
may shift." Don't use that either!

– I could put something hidden on the bottom side
of the top.

—I can't get him out of funny mode—his latest is "No b'y,
I can't." We will get the results of the MRI in an hour or so—
that'll sober us up.

At two o'clock that afternoon, Nick accompanied me and Gerry to the appointment with the radiation oncologist. We were not in our usual room, and I felt disoriented.

The oncologist came in, carrying a file in her hand. We introduced her to Nick.

"So, good news," she said, "it looks like the last radiation treatment has worked. The MRI shows just a small amount of growth."

"That's good," said Nick. Gerry nodded agreement.

She looked at us steadily. In my memory, we are standing, though that doesn't seem likely.

"So you're done now, Gerry. There's no more treatment we can offer. You don't have to come back."

This seemed impossible. What was she saying? Were they kicking us out?

"But how will he get an MRI?" I asked, puzzled.

"There won't be another MRI," she said, touching my arm. "It won't make any difference."

Up until now we had lived from MRI to MRI. It was apparent there wasn't much living left for Gerry.

"But who's going to look after him?" I said. "What about his meds, and when he gets sicker?"

She raised the file in her hand. "You'll keep being followed by the palliative care team at the Miller Centre. You've already been there."

Gerry nodded. "It'll be okay," he said to me.

"Can you tell how long he has left?" said Nick.

"I don't want to guess. There's a rule of thumb—when your

health is changing monthly, you have months, when it changes weekly, you have weeks, and when it changes daily, you have days."

"Thank you for everything," Gerry said. She gave him a hug, and then hugged Nick and me, and we said goodbye and left the building I had come to regard as our safe place. I was devastated, sad, and angry. Nick drove us home.

I went upstairs, got in bed, and cried until suppertime. No. No. No. No.

Nick came to get me.

"I've never seen you this upset," he said.

"I've probably never been this upset, before," I snuffled.

I came down to dinner in my bathrobe, red-eyed and weepy, and brought up our plans for the weekend. I was supposed to check on Heart's Content. Gerry had elected to stay home with Nick and attend a dinner party.

"You not coming to Heart's Content makes me feel like you don't love me," I said through my tears.

He tilted his head to the side. "How 'bout I change my mind?"

With a wan smile I returned to bed with a mug of tea. Gerry's baseball friends came over, and they watched the World Series. I could hear their raucous laughter through my tears.

The next morning, all three of us attended the pain and symptom management clinic at the Palliative Care Unit. We told the doctor Gerry was finding movement more difficult. Transitioning from sitting to standing left him dizzy and needing to lean on his cane. His vision was so poor, Nick and I were now describing actions on the television screen to him. "Yeah," said Gerry, "and if they get to an exciting part, they just stop talking." I laughed. "It's true," I agreed, "we're total amateurs."

The doctor went over the last MRI with us in detail and prescribed Ritalin for Gerry, to increase his energy. I told the doctor about feeling abandoned by the Cancer Centre. "I'll be with you to the end," he promised.

I know that's how the system is supposed to work. The Cancer Centre is for people who might recover or at least stay alive. Palliative care is for those who will not. But even though I'd intellectually known this would eventually happen, it was emotionally still very hard to accept that eventually was now.

After our bruising day, that night, Gerry, Nick, and I went to see Jody Sings Bowie at the Arts and Culture Centre. It was a sold-out show, with a boisterous crowd, and I was glad I had booked Gerry a seat at the end of a row, close to the stage. Nick and I sat next to him. Jody Richardson was one of the cards guys, and as he prowled the outskirts of the stage during "Jean Genie," I saw him notice Gerry. Not missing a beat, Jody leapt down and sat on Gerry's lap, singing and grinding away in his tight yellow, red, and blue one-piece. I was impressed with Gerry's quick reaction: He put his hands in the air and waved them in time to the music, laughing. Like it happened every day.

At home that night he shared his glee:

⊂⊃⊂⊃ **Gerry Porter**
@ficklesonance

Jaysus, Jody Does Bowie was as fine a show as I've ever seen. Bravo @chuckartNL. Plus. Two words, ladies: lap dance. So there.

10:46 PM – 3 Nov 2016

For me, the evening had provided a very welcome distraction. Nonetheless, the next day, I wrote this email to my friend Francine Fleming. I had been sharing the hard parts of our story with friends and family. Their support had buoyed me and kept me going.

Friday, November 4, 2016

I am pretty stressed. Tears are always close to the surface, my mind is scattered, and I have to use all my skills to keep track of what I am doing and what has to be done next. It's partly because I am still not sleeping well—I go to bed late, wake up around 4:30 a.m., and do not get back to sleep till 7:00 or so. Then I sleep in till noon!

Gerry is doing amazingly well. He is comfortable with crying when he feels like it, and a lot of his tears come in response to the love and respect being shown him by friends and colleagues. I expect we will go through boxes of tissues at Gerrypalooza!

He has about 10 per cent vision now and can't recognize anybody unless they have a really distinctive voice, so I have to stick close when we are out. Tonight he is playing cards with his poker buddies.

I think I am getting to the point where we could use meals delivered a few times a week. Could we get together and talk about that next week?

In the meantime, we were going to a Joanna Newsom tribute show, performed by Chris and Maggie and their New Music Collective. The show was a fundraiser for Girls Rock NL and had been in the works since before Gerry was diagnosed. They had decided to go ahead with it, as Gerry loved the music of Joanna Newsom, and they knew he would enjoy it.

On Saturday, November 5, Gerry, Nick, Lisa, and I joined sixty other people in the George Street United Church. We sat in the front. Chris had arranged Joanna Newsom's music for string quartet and other instruments, including piano, percussion, and harp. Maggie and other vocalists, along with eleven musicians and one dancer, performed fifteen of her songs, including Gerry's favourite, "Monkey and Bear," the source of Ursula's name. Gerry couldn't see much, but the sound in the church was soaring.

He posted about it on Twitter that night.

◯◯ **Gerry Porter**
@ficklesonance

Huge congrats to Maggie Burton and Chris McGee for the
spectacular Joanna Newsom tribute show. Holy wow.

11:32 PM - 5 Nov 2016

Only three days had passed since my meltdown over the end of
Gerry's treatment. Now the three of us went to Heart's Content for
two happy days. It was sunny, and warm enough to work outside.
I dug a new garden bed, which was deeply soothing. Following
Gerry's instructions, Nick and I successfully barbequed moose
steaks. Gerry napped, and we read to him from Stan Dragland's
new book on *The Great Eastern* radio show, *Strangers & Others*.
We even fit in some *Buffy*.

Canadian musician Leonard Cohen had been influential in
both our lives, and we mourned when he died on November 7,
reminiscing about the spectacular show we had seen him
perform in 2008. Gerry and I spent an evening sitting in the
living room, listening to his songs on YouTube. David Bowie
had liver cancer, Gord Downie had brain cancer. Problems
money can't fix, the great equalizer.

The next evening, Donald Trump was elected President of
the United States. Nick, Gerry, and I watched the results with Ed
in our living room. Gerry was vicious, although more diplomatic
about it on Twitter:

◯◯ **Gerry Porter**
@ficklesonance

Starting an existentialist polling firm specializing in "no exit" polls. Working name: Data and Nothingness.

4:26 PM - 9 Nov 2016

⌒⌒ Gerry Porter
@ficklesonance

"Star Spangled Banner" to be replaced by "Hello Darkness My Old Friend."

10:58 PM - 9 Nov 2016

⌒⌒ Gerry Porter
@ficklesonance

We live in an era where you've got to wonder if the US president will issue a racist lie today or merely hate-filled misogyny.

12:17 PM - 10 Nov 2016

A week after the Joanna Newsom show, Chris played the keyboard for a rock musical, *All Shook Up!*, which had a three-night run at the Arts and Culture Centre. Gerry and I went to see it with Maggie and Jack. We loved having a musician son.

On Remembrance Day, Gerry, a student of military history, posted:

⌒⌒ Gerry Porter
@ficklesonance

A moment to remember my late father-in-law Bob McGee, RCAF 1940–1945. A navigator on Lancaster bombers. 1/2
They were a Pathfinder squadron, which meant they flew over AA twice, once for flares, another for bombs. 2/2

11:49 PM - 11 Nov 2016

Nick made an event page on Facebook for Gerrypalooza, now a little more than two weeks away. We would invite most of the guests this way, and the ones who weren't on Facebook would be invited by email. What was needed was an eye-catching digital invitation, but Gerry's eyesight prevented him from designing it. Serendipitously, Beth, a graphic artist friend, happened to check in on us and was happy to help out.

She created a funny yet human poster, with the word *Gerrypalooza* encased in the outline of a fish. A photograph of Gerry's face was embedded, the two *O*'s of Gerrypalooza serving as the frames of his glasses. Along with the time and place were the words, "Come celebrate Gerry's life with him and his family."

I was concerned that people outside the inner circle might not understand that though Gerry would be at the party, he didn't have much time left. Under event information on Facebook, we settled on: "Gerry is not going to miss his last party. Come by and have a drink and a laugh with us."

Gerry was chuffed, posting the invitation on Twitter:

◯◯ Gerry Porter
@ficklesonance

Hey, check out the sweet invitation Beth Oberholtzer did for our pre-mortem party. Pretty funny AND civilized, we thought.

2:12 AM - 14 Nov 2016

Just two months earlier, we had been told that Gerry could be dead by now. But with an event to plan, we both felt a renewed energy. It might be a pre-mortem party, but damn it, Gerrypalooza was going to be fun!

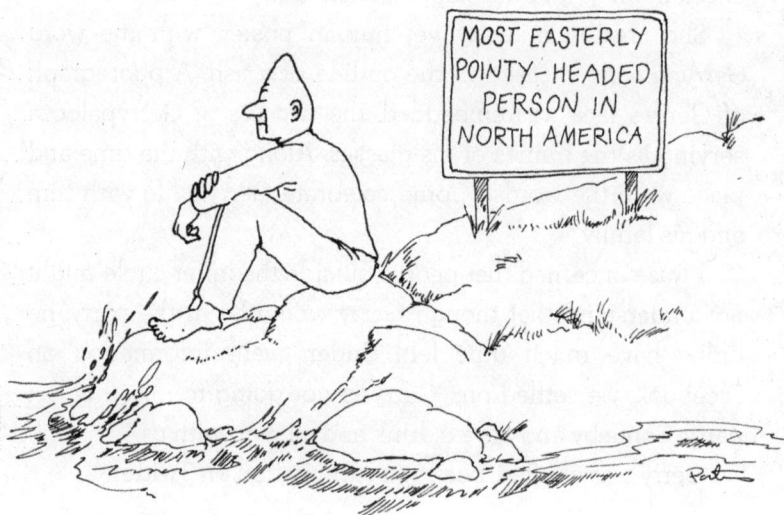

MOST EASTERLY
POINTY-HEADED
PERSON IN
NORTH AMERICA

ʃIX

August 19, 1987. The baby passed the birth inspection and was delivered back to me on the maternity ward. He was tiny—five pounds, fifteen ounces. I decided to name him Nicholas Robert McGee. When my doctor came to see us, I told her I had dim memories of making a huge racket during birth.

"Keep them dim," she replied.

In 1987, women remained longer in hospital after giving birth, and I had a fair bit of healing to do. We would stay there for almost a week.

The day after the birth, Lois called, masquerading as my sister. "Gerry would like to see the baby," she told me.

Of course he would. As much as I knew Vernon was not going to like this, I felt it could be important to the baby's future psychology to know his biological father had been interested enough to see him at birth.

"Okay. Not today, though. He can come tomorrow," I said.

Lying in the hospital bed, I told this to Vernon, knowing in advance how he would react.

"This is a deal-breaker," Vernon shouted. "If he comes, I am leaving!" As he yelled, I repeated my position, each time in a weaker voice. "It's not for Gerry, it's for the baby." I was so exhausted, I thought I might pass out. Could a new mother die from stress? I wonder now why no one came to check on what was happening. Maybe men yelling in hospital rooms was normal in those days. I like to think that in today's world, a security detail would have come hurtling in.

After all the drama, the next day a mutual friend took Vernon for lunch, while Lois accompanied Gerry to the hospital. Nicholas had developed infant jaundice, and Gerry could only see him through the glass walls of an incubator. Gerry and I did not meet.

The birth of the baby changed things. I had someone who needed me to look out for them, and there just wasn't time for neurosis. It also marked the end of my journal-keeping. The first week home at The Terrace, I crawled from the bed where I still spent most of my time and, sitting at my PC Jr. computer while the baby napped, managed to write a lengthy account of the birth and my time in hospital. Exhausted, I turned off the computer without hitting the save button. Much of what I'd written was gone. I knew immediately I would not try again.

Vernon was able to stay another two weeks. He was smitten with baby Nicholas, taking countless photographs. Any worries I had about him loving the baby disappeared. He wanted to wear the Snugli, give the baths, change the diapers. All was well.

I imagine having a baby in the house was somewhat disruptive to my roommates, Ange and Evelyn. I didn't give it much thought, since we had all known for a while that this would be happening. I didn't expect them to change their ways because of the baby, and I wasn't worried about the baby upsetting the household rhythm, which had always been flexible.

In mid-September, Vernon left to get prepped for his shoot. I remained, slowly healing, thrilled with my baby, receiving cards and letters, happily visiting with friends bringing me presents, and nursing constantly. By his four-week checkup, Nick had gained three pounds. He had a cold, a rash, and an eye infection. My doctor was calm, I was anxious, and the baby unperturbed.

Two weeks later, at the beginning of October, I flew to Toronto to stay with Vernon before his departure for Europe, planned for later that month. Nick was six weeks old. Vernon was now living in a house I found questionable, just off Queen Street near a chicken slaughterhouse. He had painted the room before our arrival but hadn't cleaned up the painting tools, nor put the room back in order. I was truly shocked. My tiny, perfect baby should not be sleeping in the presence of open paint cans and wet rollers. What was Vernon thinking? I kept imagining what my father would say, something along the lines of, "This is just not done."

Poor Vernon was shocked at my distress. He had been expecting to get some support from me as he prepared for his film shoot, but I was busy 24-7 with the baby, and when I took a break, it was to devour my copy of *Your Baby and Child, from Birth to Age Five,* by baby guru Penelope Leach.

I stayed in Toronto for two weeks. My sisters Robin and Jan were attending the University of Western Ontario and came up from London to see their nephew. Vernon and I visited friends to show off the baby. One day when I was home alone with Nicholas, the phone rang. It was Sue, the woman Vernon had been seeing before we got together. He had characterized her as neurotic, a needy friend who wouldn't leave him alone.

"Did you know Vernon was seeing me these past months? You should leave him. You can't trust him."

I brushed off her concerns. I did in fact have doubts, but I had made my bed and wasn't going to leave it easily. Instead, we planned that Nicholas and I would join Vernon in Amsterdam, which was his station for the shoot.

When Vernon left for Europe in mid-October, Nick and I took the train to Ottawa to stay with my parents, a soothing balm. Mom and Dad were anxious for things to work out for me. A few weeks later, they drove us to Mirabel International Airport, where we took a flight to London and met up with Vernon.

We arrived in Amsterdam in the second week of November, to the teeniest apartment in the world. It was like living in a boat— the kitchen a galley, with storage compartments cleverly built inside every wooden surface. I made Nick a crib in my suitcase, placed on the floor next to the pull-out bed. Vernon was frantic about the shoot, I was having an allergic reaction to penicillin, and Nick cried a lot and wouldn't sleep. It would have been a hellish experience, except we were in Amsterdam. The city was enchanting: networked canals, arched bridges, narrow cobblestone streets, tall colourful houses, and windmills! Vernon expected me to provide home-base support, I expected him to spell me off when he returned from work. What had I been thinking? Every time Vernon raged (not necessarily at me), I would consider calling it quits and going home—but we were in Amsterdam. People seemed to love babies; in every store and restaurant, Nicholas was deluged with attention. Vernon, Nick, and I went to the Rijksmuseum and saw the Rembrandts and Vermeers, the Van Gogh Museum, and Anne Frank House. We took a day trip to see the ground reclaimed from the Zuiderzee by a thirty-two-kilometre dyke, and stopped on the way back for supper, my first taste of venison. We even went for a sad walk around the red-light district, where the smell of cannabis filled the air. Despite everything, it was interesting. And I was still not willing to admit, even to myself, that maybe I'd made a mistake.

At the end of November, with the film shoot finished and our relationship strained, one of Vernon's old friends, now a wealthy restaurateur in Copenhagen, insisted on treating Vernon and me to a visit in London. It was a few weeks before Christmas, and the city was done up in lights. We stayed with him and his partner in a modern hotel, ate in nice restaurants, and met their old friends for curry—but my biggest memory is of Vernon looking over his shoulder at us as he prepared to step off the curb, not realizing he was steering the baby stroller into two lanes of oncoming traffic. Thank goodness our horrified shouts stopped him in time.

That was a turning point for me. Vernon loved Nicholas, adored him. But from then on, I didn't trust him with the baby's safety. How could I call myself a responsible mother if I chose to have an irresponsible father? It was time to concede I knew Vernon had major issues and stop naively hoping that love would conquer all.

Nick and I had now been in Europe for almost six weeks. We all returned to Canada together, flying from London directly to Ottawa for a pleasant Christmas with my family. We stayed with my parents for one week (in separate bedrooms) and then house-sat a friend's apartment downtown for a week.

After New Year's I went home to The Terrace for six weeks, and Vernon returned to Toronto. It wasn't easy having a baby and no car in downtown St. John's in winter. But I finally had time to reflect. I read a self-help book called *Men Who Hate Women and the Women Who Love Them*. I felt it described my situation with Vernon. Jealousy, temper tantrums, drinking—it was time to set boundaries.

My film budget allowed me to return to Toronto, where my friend Petra was going to edit my film, which had been sitting at NIFCO since September. We would work at the National Film Board offices. Nick and I would stay with my brother David, who had an extra room in his apartment in the Annex. No way I was going back to the chicken slaughterhouse.

Before I left St. John's, I ran into Gerry and Mary on Water Street. Nick was asleep in the Snugli. We all stopped to talk. Feeling kindly disposed, I asked if he wanted to see the baby. Mary discreetly moved to window-shop while I lifted the flannel receiving blanket and Gerry gazed at Nick's sleeping face. He was perfection. I said I was leaving soon for Toronto. Gerry nodded. We went our separate ways. I felt gracious, even mature.

I arrived in Toronto on Valentine's Day. Leaving the baby with my brother, Vernon and I went out for dinner, where I began the difficult conversation at the restaurant table. He had to be less possessive and drop his phobia about Gerry and the baby. Gerry did not provide financial support. I rarely saw him, and he rarely saw the baby, but Vernon behaved as if I spent all my time in St. John's facilitating visits. His position was that no card, no letter, not the most minute gift should ever come to Nicholas from Gerry. Despite my distaste for Gerry, I insisted that the best thing for Nicholas would be to know his biological father, or at the very least, know of him. I would not lie to my child. It was an impasse, and we agreed to seek counselling.

It took a while to get an appointment. In the intervening weeks, Nick and I spent most of our days at the NFB, where Petra was working hard. Finally, the film was picture-edited. Vernon, who was staying with us at my brother's apartment, was enthusiastic about the cut, arranging for me to show it to a few of his influential film contacts.

At last Vernon and I went for counselling. It was an evening appointment, and we walked up the pathway of a private house in the Annex and knocked on the wooden front door. Our counsellor, a middle-aged woman, greeted us and showed us to her basement office.

To say the session went badly is an understatement. In my memory, I see Vernon standing, shouting as he threatened that this would be the end of our relationship. I held to my position. His anger was frightening, and I was glad we were having the discussion in the presence of another person and that the baby was with my brother. The counsellor seemed much more sympathetic to Vernon's position than to mine. At the end of our appointment, the counsellor stated, "Unless one of you changes your mind, I don't see any future in this relationship." I returned to St. John's and The Terrace a few days later, around the beginning of April, baby and suitcase of film in hand, unsure of my next steps. Nick was almost eight months old.

Vernon was contemplating moving from Toronto to BC, his original home. I had no desire to join him. My film needed sound editing, and that could be done at NIFCO. I decided that for the time being, Nick and I would be better off staying in St. John's.

But living in The Terrace was not going to be viable for Nicholas and me much longer. We needed more space and more control of the environment. I started looking for a permanent place for us to live. In 1988, many of us in the St. John's arts community lived by hiring each other for ten weeks, using money from our project grants, and then applying for unemployment insurance. I had to be budget conscious, but I could afford to live on my own.

Once again, NIFCO came to my rescue. At the time, NIFCO owned two adjoining houses, 40 and 42 King's Road, and one of them had an apartment on the top two floors. It was four blocks from The Hall and five blocks from The Ship. The current tenants were moving out, and I moved in on July 1. Nick was ten months old.

The apartment was palatial. There was a large kitchen, a living room, two bedrooms, and a small office. It even had a laundry room. I borrowed couches for the living room, bought lamps from a thrift store, got a second-hand washing machine and dryer, and began to develop a small stable of babysitters.

I remember a housewarming party at the apartment, where I received much needed pots and pans. I remember looking out the living room window, watching the crowds from NIFCO arrive and depart on various film shoots. Summer trolled along. I was often lonely, at home with just the baby.

Using a baby monitor, I began to work in the night at NIFCO. The apartment had its own street entrance, but it was possible to enter NIFCO from the apartment staircase via a door that had been created on the first-floor landing. Working in the upstairs editing room, there was only one wall separating me from Nick's room. If I heard him wake up, I could run down the NIFCO stairs, through the adjoining door, and dash up the stairs to my apartment.

Sometime in July, working at NIFCO one evening, another filmmaker said to me, "Gerry would really like to be part of Nick's life."

"No he wouldn't," I scoffed. "All Gerry cares about is Mary."

She looked baffled. But from my point of view, he seemed to have no interest in Nick. He had never once contacted me since I returned to St. John's in April. His sister, Lisa, had more initiative. She had asked a couple of months earlier if she could take Nicholas to visit her mother once a week, and I was happy to agree. She had a car, I lent her Nick's car seat, and I felt Nick would be safe with his aunt and grandmother.

On our phone calls, Vernon was talking more and more about moving to Vancouver. I had no interest in returning there and was ambivalent about the relationship with Vernon. But when Vernon's mother offered to pay for our trip, I agreed to a ten-day visit in mid-July. The first stop was Qualicum Beach on Vancouver Island.

Vernon's mother was very welcoming to me and Nicholas. The weather was beautiful, all blue sky and towering mountains, and we made sandcastles on the sandy beach as the waves rolled in.

The night before we left, Vernon's brother came to visit. It was a lovely summer evening, and the two of them sat on camp chairs in the driveway, talking and drinking. I went to bed and was awakened by Vernon entering the room. He was completely drunk, so drunk that he peed in a corner, and then stumbled out. I was aghast. Nicholas was sleeping. I got up cautiously. Vernon had just missed peeing in the baby's suitcase. I had no idea it was possible for someone to get that drunk. It frightened me. I knew I did not want that in my baby's life.

We took the Nanaimo ferry to Vancouver, where I introduced Nicholas to my film and school friends. It had been almost three years since I moved to St. John's, and much had changed for me. A new film and a new baby, but not, apparently, a new love. When Nicholas and I returned home, I knew it was for good.

Looking back, I am astonished by my eighteen-month relationship with Vernon. Certainly, attitudes have changed since then as to what is acceptable. I think because I didn't feel physically threatened, I never once thought I was in an abusive relationship. Yes, he was emotionally volatile. Yes, he had a drinking problem. At the time, that described half the men in my community and a quarter of the women. I was so in love with Vernon and so committed to working through our issues that it took my concerns over the baby to finally move me to action. It gives me new insight into the many news articles I have read on domestic violence, shaking my head, wondering "why she stayed." I see now from my own life experience why some women stay: because when it's good, it can be very good, and because when lives become enmeshed, it is very hard to untangle them. Thank you, women's movement and feminist activists everywhere, for helping to change the norms, though there is still a long way to go.

It was now early August. I bought a TV and a VCR, necessities for someone spending a lot of time alone with a child. *General Hospital* and *Sesame Street* became my new best friends. I had applied for a grant from the Linda Joy Busby Foundation, stating I would use the money for babysitting, which would allow me to finish the film in the daytime. The grant came through, as did one for music composition from the Newfoundland and Labrador Arts Council.

Ange, my old roommate from The Terrace, told me she was dating Gerry, and she hoped I didn't mind. I certainly didn't. I was just happy to know that Mary was no longer in the picture.

On August 19, Nicholas had his first birthday, celebrated with an afternoon party in our apartment, attended by my friends and anyone I knew who had a child or baby. Nick was now walking and had a small vocabulary, consisting of words like "broccoli" and "tasty." Lisa, who had now taken Nicholas on several occasions, phoned me.

"Would it be alright if Gerry and I stopped by? He wants to give Nick a birthday gift."

I hadn't been in the same room as Gerry in months, and it was bound to be awkward. But it was in line with my philosophy of Nicholas knowing his father. I agreed.

They arrived in the late afternoon and came into the sunny living room, where Nick was sitting on the carpet, playing with wooden blocks. He immediately went over to offer them his two purple triangles. "Those are very nice," said Gerry, taking one in his hand.

We made small talk. Gerry was currently working on a one-year contract as a graphic designer for the student union at Memorial University. "Next month, I'm starting a permanent job at MUN Extension," he said.

"As a graphic artist?" I asked.

"No, as an information and publications officer."

I was impressed that Gerry was stable enough to have a real job, with real benefits. But mostly I was impressed by how well Nick got along with him. I had seen Nick with many strangers, and while he was not particularly shy, he and Gerry seemed to have a bond. Did Nick recognize his genetic material? This softened me toward Gerry in a way that nothing else could have.

It never occurred to me that they *did* know each other. I found out later that Gerry had been going to his mother's every time Nicholas was there.

Gerry seemed to have changed. I didn't know what he had gone through in the eighteen months since we had separated, but he seemed older, more mature. He lived just a few blocks away. I can't recall how it happened, but slowly Gerry began to help me out—the first time on a rainy day when I called to ask him to stay with thirteen-month-old Nicholas while I filled a prescription for his ear infection.

Soon, Gerry was coming by on a regular basis to see Nick. Sometimes on a weekend he would take Nick to Bannerman Park, only a few blocks away. I watched as he helped Nick put his little arms into his turquoise jacket, then button it up, all the while talking gently. "Are you going to the park? What do you think you'll do there?"

On the film front, hiring a regular babysitter allowed me to start working during the day. I learned how to sound edit, greatly aided by a visiting film editor from Halifax. She showed me how to lay out the tracks and do the charts for a sound mix. This occupied me for all of September.

Vernon moved to Vancouver. Things were amiable between us. We both knew our relationship had run its course. He was probably as relieved as I was.

In October of 1988, MUN Extension Services offered me a four-month contract editing five videos for the Rural Women's Leadership Project, run out of their offices at the university. It would interfere with working on my own film, but I figured I had the rest of my life to be a successful filmmaker. In the meanwhile, I didn't want to turn down the money or the experience of learning video editing. Gerry and I began sharing cabs to and from work. My editing room was on the first floor of the Extension building on campus, and Gerry's office was on the floor above. We didn't see each other much during the day, as our jobs were quite separate, but he would stop in to see Nick in the morning or after work, and I continued to be impressed by how well they got along.

Gerry was tender, solicitous, and engaged, not to mention patient, with Nick. Sometimes he would stay for supper and afterwards give Nick a bath. They developed a routine, based on a skit from *Sesame Street*. Gerry would help Nick line up his "guys," small figures of people, dogs, and animals on the side of the bathtub. Nick would pour bath water from a white plastic cup into a yellow plastic cup, then carefully place a figure in it, offering it to Gerry, saying "Jure soup" in his high-pitched voice. "I'd love some soup du jour," Gerry would reply, and then pretend to sip it. Nick would sit back in the tub, his face bright with anticipation, waiting for Gerry to say, "Hey, wait a minute! Waiter, there's a puppy dog in my soup. I can't eat this." Nick, always delighted, would say, "I bwing back." Then there would be another round.

I loved Nick so much, and it was clear to me that Gerry did too. Could we be partners again?

Once this thought had entered my mind, I couldn't shake it. I developed a crush on Gerry, which I carefully hid. I recall watching him come down the stairs at work, and thinking he was the cutest thing I had ever seen, with his curly auburn hair and slim body. Or noticing his dark chest-hair peeking out of his loose-fitting shirts, tucked into his belted cargo pants. I suppose it didn't hurt that I had happy memories of our sex life.

I determined that I was going to propose to Gerry that we get back together. I wanted to do this before Ange returned from Labrador, where she had gone to run a campaign for the New Democratic Party.

The country was in the middle of a federal election, and Gerry and I often watched the coverage together on my new television. The campaign was being fought over free trade with the United States, and it seemed likely that the Conservative Mulroney government would win over John Turner's Liberals. It was a depressing time for political progressives, and I told Gerry my theory that the best hope for change lay with Indigenous Peoples and their increasing militancy and resistance.

Election Day was on November 21, 1988. I took the day off work to volunteer as a zone captain for Jack Harris, our NDP Member of Parliament. Gerry looked after Nick that evening, and when I returned after the polls closed, we sat together on the old brown-plaid couch in my living room, watching the election results together. It was a landslide victory for the Conservatives. Jack Harris was defeated. I was disappointed but not depressed, having been part of many losing campaigns since my first one in 1974.

And I had my own campaign to run. Ange would soon return from Labrador. It was now or never. I turned down the volume on the television.

"Gerry, could I talk to you about something?"

"Sure." He picked up his Old Stock beer.

"We've spent a lot of time together, and I'm becoming quite fond of you. I was wondering if you might be interested in getting back together."

He choked mid-swallow. "You mean, as a couple?"

"Yes."

He put the bottle down and sat up straight on the couch. He had to think, he said.

"And I have to talk to Ange about this, first."

"Yes, of course." I was happy to hear that. Ange was my friend, too.

"She's coming home tomorrow. I'll come over after I speak with her."

"Yes, of course," I said again.

We were careful to give each other a wide berth as he gathered his coat to leave. The next evening, he returned after Nick was in bed. Gerry sat down on the tattered couch, and I sat across the room on a lumpy beige armchair. The dark brown rug seemed as wide as an ocean. The atmosphere was strangely formal, no music, no television. He cleared his throat.

"I told Ange that we're going to try and make this work. She's okay with it."

I nodded.

"But if we are to do this, I would want to move in, within six months."

"Yes."

"And we would have to put the past behind us. No bringing up of who did what to whom."

"Agreed."

We didn't shake hands, but I referred to this ever after as our Terms of Union meeting.

I was ecstatic. For the first time in a long time, I had no doubts. I wanted this.

I moved to sit beside him, and we awkwardly embraced. Within seconds, we were kissing passionately, and I remember his surprised laugh as I pressed him down on the couch.

———

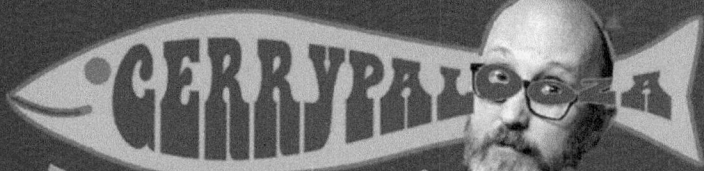

Come celebrate **GERRY**'s life with him *&* his family

GERRY

GERRYPALOOZA

NOV 25 • 7-10 PM

at the ROCKET ROOM   272 Water Street   St. John's

SEVEN

Gerrypalooza was two weeks away, and it seemed Gerry was likely to make it. Although we knew he didn't have long, it seemed the secondary radiation had given him more time. Gerry hoped to make it through Christmas, saying, "I don't want to wreck everyone's holiday."

But as his eyesight and physical energy declined, the activities of daily life, such as getting washed, dressed, and up and down the stairs to the bathroom were taking more and more time. Shopping and cooking were falling by the wayside. We were ready for help on the food front.

Thursday, November 10, 2016

Dear Friends,

You are receiving this email because at some point you either offered to, or did, help out Gerry and me with food. We have been managing fairly well this summer and fall, but now things are getting to the point where we pretty much rely on takeout. So once again we turn to the community. Please don't feel any pressure—personal situations change and you can't do everything.

The wonderful Francine Fleming, who is copied on this email, has volunteered to take on the task of organizing food assistance for us. She will be contacting you to see if you are available, and she will have the information you need. Also, if you know someone who would like to get involved, please ask them to contact Francine.

Thank you so much.

Debbie and Gerry

Francine, a consummate organizer, soon had three weeks of meals arranged. She provided us with a schedule to show the menu for each night and who was bringing it. It was humbling to see the names of friends, family members, and even acquaintances who had signed on to provide luxury meals. "I feel warm and fuzzy with all the kind offers," I told Francine. The first meal drop-off was on November 14, pot roast with lots of root vegetables, a rhubarb/strawberry crisp, and a bottle of red wine.

Gerry had continued to post his ire about the election of Donald Trump on social media, but as we got closer to Gerrypalooza, he found some time for events closer to home.

👓 **Gerry Porter**
@ficklesonance

Delegation from the family heading down to the Rocket to sort out food and booze. Gerrypalooza is happening, people!

3:08 PM - 17 Nov 2016

I fervently hoped that nothing would happen to derail the event. Each day Gerry was weaker. On November 18, an occupational therapist from the community health palliative care team made a home visit, examining our bathroom situation. We had two. There was a small ensuite off our bedroom, with a stacked washer-dryer, a two-shelf unit covered in plants in front of the window, a toilet, and a round shower stall. Add in our clothes cupboard, and there was barely room to turn around. The larger bathroom at the end of the upstairs hallway had a bathtub, which Gerry was now using with assistance from me or Nick. The OT had suggestions for installing grab bars for the tub, which Gerry approved. Nick and I privately felt it was too late for that. Gerry was not strong enough to hoist himself anywhere, no matter how many grab bars were available. The OT also provided us with a commode, in case we needed it later.

Our friend Susan Shiner checked in with us, and I texted her back:

November 18, 2016, 3:47 p.m.

—Gerry is spending a lot of the day in bed now. The stairs are very energy-draining and getting to be a safety issue. Nick and I continue to work on Gerrypalooza. I have four relatives coming from Ontario for it, and Gerry has five, and I am beginning to realize our hosting duties will extend well beyond the actual party. Gulp.
Tonight, there is a launch for Stan Dragland's book on the Great Eastern radio show. It's at the Crow's Nest! How we are going to get Gerry up there is beyond me. Best advice so far, "start early." XOXO

The Crow's Nest Officers' Club is across from the harbour, at the top of a steep staircase on the outside of a tall building near the St. John's War Memorial. Stan Dragland's book launch for *Strangers & Others: The Great Eastern* would take place there at seven-thirty. As the volunteer graphic artist and the "official" unofficial archivist and webmaster for the CBC Radio show *The Great Eastern*, and as someone named in the book, Gerry very much wanted to be there with his pals Ed Riche, Steve Palmer, and Mack Furlong, the show's creators. Nick and I plotted a course of action. We had a gift certificate for Pi, a restaurant across the street from the Crow's Nest, given to us by our friend Joan, who did not like to cook but wanted to participate in feeding us. If we ate at five-thirty, we could arrive in time for the book launch and avoid heading up a winding conga-line of fellow guests waiting for us to slowly ascend to the top.

All during our supper of pizza and salad, Gerry was planning his remarks. He wanted to complain about CBC management and how they refused to participate in archiving *The Great Eastern*. He knew his pals from the show did not want to air this grievance publicly, so he was of two minds about what to say. After settling the bill, we slowly crossed Duckworth Street and headed to the infamous staircase. It took almost twenty minutes to climb the fifty-nine steps, me beside Gerry and his cane, and Nick behind him. All of us were exhausted when we arrived at the Crow's Nest.

Entering the Crow's Nest is like stepping back into the time of the Second World War. One end of the room has a tall brick fireplace, overhung with a wooden helm and a brass ship's bell. Thick dark-brown posts support the slanted ceiling. Every wall is covered with maritime artifacts from the Battle of the Atlantic, including colourful gun-shield art from wartime naval vessels, ship badges, oil paintings, photographs, and all manner of model ships encased in glass. A periscope from a German U-boat rises through the ceiling and can be used to scan St. John's Harbour. No wonder the Crow's Nest is a National Historic Site.

We wended our way through the armchairs and tables and sat on a dilapidated maroon leather couch near the fireplace. I went to the large wooden bar on the opposite wall and returned with draft beer for Nick and Gerry. I wasn't going to drink until it felt safe to relax. Soon the room was crowded with thirty to forty fans of both Stan Dragland and *The Great Eastern*. I was on the other side of the room when it was Gerry's turn to speak. He stood to talk, leaning on his cane, and Nick rose too, standing beside Gerry, looking like an interpreter but needing to be there in case his father lost his balance. Gerry hesitated at the beginning, and apprehensive that he might not be able to continue, I began strategizing on how best to intervene. But soon Gerry began speaking and acquitted himself well with brief remarks about the pleasures of maintaining the *Great Eastern* archival website and only a tiny dig at the CBC. He got a round of applause. I got a drink.

We left around ten o'clock. Somehow, with the help of a few friends, we all made it back down the stairs alive. Nick went ahead to get the car and brought it as close as possible to where Gerry and I waited on the sidewalk. We couldn't afford any more of these energy-draining nights if Gerry was going to make it to Gerrypalooza.

Gerrypalooza was now less than a week away. Lisa and I were planning the family component, and I texted her:

November 19, 2016, 10:29 p.m.

—Do you have a breakdown of when the Huntley cousins
arrive and leave?

—Thursday to Monday. Don't know flight times. Will ask.

—I know everybody will want to spend time with Gerry. Trying to figure out how to make that happen without exhausting him. Maybe scheduled showings, like with the Dionne quintuplets!

—Hahaha

I continued to wake in the night, with a feeling I recognized as anxiety. I couldn't take the sleeping pills my doctor had prescribed, as they left me too groggy to drive. None of my calming techniques worked. Adrenalin coursed through me, as my mind leapt to planning and worrying. One night I reached out my hand, placing it on Gerry as he slept, and instantly felt grounded. I fell asleep.

Gerry's playlist for Gerrypalooza was not yet finished. As his vision decreased, it had become difficult for him to work on it. Now Nick was helping him. The Tuesday night before Gerrypalooza found us all sitting in the office, Nick and Gerry working on the playlist at his computer. Three feet away, I was preparing an illustrated history of Gerry's life on PowerPoint at my computer and responding to his questions on the playlist.

"Do you want some Donovan? Which one?" Gerry asked.

"Oh yes, Donovan!" I said. "How about 'Season of the Witch' or 'Sunshine Superman'?"

"Let's have both."

That night, Gerry made his last post on Facebook:

🎧 **Gerry Porter**
November 22, 2016

I guess if you were devising a Newfoundland-specific political vocabulary, it would have to include "right honourable, b'ye."

The next day, Wednesday, November 23, the doctor from the PCU at the Miller Centre came by for a home visit. He assessed Gerry's ability to stand from a sitting position and a tremor in his hands and feet and agreed it was time for a wheelchair. I arranged to pick one up the next day from a nearby medical supply store. In the afternoon, Gerry's father and his partner, Jill, arrived for Gerrypalooza, again staying with Lisa. Nick had an appointment to see the counsellor at the Miller Centre, pronouncing it helpful when he returned home.

As for Gerry, he was still making jokes about Canadian politics. This tweet references the Special Committee on Electoral Reform and the referendum that Justin Trudeau had promised on moving Canada to a system of proportional representation.

ᗢᗒ **Gerry Porter**
@ficklesonance
Electoral reform debates expected to spell the end of democracy in Canada.
3:05 PM - 23 Nov 2016

As I found out later, it was the last time Gerry posted on Twitter. Even though he was unsteady on his feet, Gerry wanted to attend that evening's launch of John Doyle's book *Riddle Me This One: A Treasury of Newfoundland Trivia*. Gerry had been at home all day and had taken Ritalin, which gave him the energy he needed to go out. So after our supper delivery of roast chicken and vegetables, at six o'clock Nick, Gerry, and I, as well as Paul, Lisa, Gerry Sr., and Jill, went to the book launch at a piano bar on

Water Street. Gerry enjoyed the event but had to remain in his seat, while people came to chat with him. We got home by eight o'clock, as Nick had to pick up Caitlin at the airport.

The next day, the last before Gerrypalooza, I picked up the wheelchair, a case of wine, and my sister Gail and brother Mark from the airport. I took them to their B&B on Monkstown Road, just around the corner from us, and relaxed while they compared rooms and jousted over the best one. Sitting on the bed in Gail's room, I explained to them how precarious Gerry's health was. "You'll be surprised when you see him, Gail. He can't see anymore and has a hard time standing, even with his cane. I'm so glad Gerrypalooza is tomorrow, 'cause I don't think he'd be able to do it next week." My voice shook a little. I could see their faces sober as they realized how close he was to the end. "Anyway," I continued, "we'll see you tonight at our house."

We had invited all the out-of-town family to come over for a drink that evening. Lisa had arranged for their cousins Alison and Lorraine to stay with a friend on Monkstown Road, only a block from our house. My two siblings were introduced to Gerry's two cousins by Lisa and Paul, who, of course, knew them all. All four of them, as well as Gerry Sr. and Jill, met Caitlin for the first time. Everyone sat in the living room, serving themselves wine from the kitchen and munching on nibblies. Gerry enjoyed himself hugely. I could hear his laugh as Nick and I sat in the office next door, feverishly working on our presentations for Gerrypalooza. Less than twenty-four hours to go! After the guests left around ten, I helped Gerry into the office, and he sat beside me at my computer as I read him my speech, describing the photos to go with each section.

"Are you okay with that?" I asked.

He nodded. "Yes. I like it," he said.

The next morning there were many wheels in motion, people delivering items to the Rocket Room, texts flying back and forth. The to-do list on my phone for the day reads:

Coat racks and hangers
Music onto iPod
PowerPoint onto MacPro
Posters to Paul
Info to Chris – award
Lasagna Sat.
Check slideshow
Practice presentation
Pens
Memorial sign-in book
3M hooks
Gerry bath
Gerry clothes
Polish shoes
Second reminder to sign book
Thanks to Francine and the food support friends
Gerry's music playing

I was getting excited. I wanted this to go well. Our workmates from MUN would bring and set up the projectors and the sound. Except for during the speeches, Gerry's posters and artwork would be projected continuously, while his playlist would provide music.

Brother-in-law Paul had taken charge of collecting mounted posters of Gerry's work. There were about thirty of them, in a variety of sizes and colours, and a team had been assembled to hang them around the Rocket Room.

The Room was on the top floor and could be entered by a staircase or through a back-door ramp. The plan was that as guests came up the staircase, they would pass through an entry room, where my friend Elaine Wychreschuk would invite them to hang their coats, sign the guest book, and help themselves to a complimentary drink ticket. From there they would enter the main room, with its vaulted wooden ceiling and tall rectangular windows. A stage and screen were set up in the front of the room, with the bar and the food tables at the opposite end, near the back door.

There would be speeches from me, Nick, and Chris. I had also asked Ed Riche to speak, as he was Gerry's best friend since childhood, and actor Charlie Tomlinson, a friend of us both, to be the MC.

My brother Jim and his wife, Debbie, arrived from Ottawa in the afternoon. They were staying at the same B&B as Gail and Mark, a fifteen-minute walk from the Rocket Room.

In the late afternoon I gave Gerry a bath, apologizing for having been so busy. "When this is over, I'm going to stay home all next week, and we can just hang out."

But now I headed down to the Rocket to make sure everything was going according to plan. It was indeed. The screen was up on the red brick wall behind the stage, and the MUN team began testing the slide presentation and music playlist on my laptop. Paul was supervising the hanging of Gerry's posters, being careful not to damage the white walls.

Nick had made two signs to be placed in strategic places. They featured the cut-out of Gerry from the invitation delivering the following message:

Hello there!

Thanks for coming to the party!
I can't see you
very well, so please
announce yourself
to me with first and last names
when you come say hi.
That way I know
who I'm talking to.
Thanks!

I placed one on the entry wall of the staircase and the other on the table beside the sign-in book. Soon, all was ready, and the group of us chatted and snacked as we awaited the arrival of guests. We watched the Rocket staff as they set up the first food service on the tables at the back: four dozen each of salt cod cakes, Moroccan meatballs with tzatziki, tomato herb and parmesan tartlets, vegetarian *gougères*, and polenta with chipotle, roasted sweet potato, and cilantro pesto. There was also a large fresh fruit tray, a hummus and fresh baked bread tray, and forty assorted desserts. We were expecting at least 150 people, and I wanted to be sure there was enough food to go round and that vegans, vegetarians, and gluten-sensitive guests would find something to eat.

Back at home, Caitlin had picked up Gerry's favourite take-out, the daily special from International Flavours, and Nick had helped his father dress in a spiffy new blue-checked shirt. Gerrypalooza officially began at seven o'clock, and there were already about forty people at the party by the time Gerry arrived in his wheelchair, escorted through the back door by Nick and Caitlin.

Guests were enjoying drinks and holding plates of food, listening to the playlist and remarking on the slideshow. I was shocked when I noticed Gerry standing without his cane, chatting with the group of men I called "the cards guys."

"It must be the testosterone keeping him upright," I said to Paul.

The cards guys had been playing poker together for over thirty years and were like the arts version of Fight Club—the first rule of cards is that you don't talk about cards. As a result, I didn't know much about what went on at cards, except that they held an elaborate Christmas game every year, eating a huge and hugely expensive cut of beef on bread rolls. I also knew Gerry loved playing cards, and I was deeply grateful for all the pleasure it had given him over the past months.

A short while later, Gerry was leaning on his cane, and soon he was safe in his wheelchair.

Jack and Ursula enjoyed the people, the snacks, and until it became too crowded, the ability to run up and down the room, climbing on and off the stage. The speeches were scheduled for eight o'clock, and when it was time to begin, I gave Charlie the pre-arranged signal.

"There's something else first," he said.

"What do you mean, something else first?" I said indignantly. "I'm organizing this!"

But unbeknownst to us, Peg Norman had organized a group of people, who over the last few days had been rehearsing a song chosen by Lisa. Guitars and a cajon drum suddenly appeared. Lyric sheets courtesy of Maggie Keiley were passed out. Soon over 150 people were singing The Talking Heads' "Road to Nowhere," and all the love and concern and bewilderment at what had befallen their dear friend was expressed in their heartfelt singing. It was the community in action.

Road to Nowhere

Well, we know where we're going
But we don't know where we've been
And we know what we're knowing
But we can't say what we've seen
And we're not little children
And we know what we want
And the future is certain
Give us time to work it out

Yeah

We're on a road to nowhere
Come on inside
Taking that ride to nowhere
We'll take that ride
I'm feeling okay this morning
And you know
We're on the road to paradise
Here we go, here we go

The video of the song shows Gerry in his wheelchair, flanked by me, lyric sheet in hand. I bend down to speak in his ear a few times, telling him things like "Chris is playing guitar" or "Ursula has climbed on the stage." Gerry is smiling, nodding to the rhythm with a glass of red wine in his hand, touched and delighted, sometimes singing along. The camera pans across the room. Most are singing whole-heartedly, especially Lisa, but the odd few are solemnly gazing around, absorbing this extraordinary moment. Some appear to be focused on suppressing tears. At the end of the song, two women friends bend over to kiss Gerry's forehead.

After the applause and cheering died down, Charlie introduced me and I stepped up on the stage. My words were illustrated with a PowerPoint presentation of photographs and images, which I could control from the laptop on the podium in front of me, often causing raucous outbursts of laughter or fervent applause. Gerry, still holding his red wine, sat with Lisa to the side of the stage next to me, turned so they could view the screen. At the front of the room, guests sat on the floor, while behind them, crowded rows of people stood, watching. I felt very comfortable as I held the microphone in my hand and began.

> *Thank you so much for being here with us tonight. You have all been great. Now that I'm up here, I keep seeing people I haven't hugged yet. It's amazing how many people are here.*
>
> *One of the black jokes that we've been making over the past six months is: While St. John's is a great place to live in, it's an even better place to die in.* [scandalized laughter]
>
> *And on that note, I'd like to do a special shout-out to Francine Fleming and our food support team. You guys are literally lifesavers.* [applause]
>
> *Tonight, although it's not easy to summarize fifty-four years of a life, I'm going to attempt to do just that, with an illustrated look at the life of Gerald Cameron Porter.*

A baby picture of Gerry and his mom appeared on the screen, to laughter and applause.

> *Gerry Porter was born on September 12, 1962, to the very beautiful and very cool Ida Healey Porter and the very cool*

Gerry Porter—well, I call him "Senior."

"Big Gerry," a voice called out. "We call him Big Gerry."

That's right, Big Gerry and Little Gerry, that's how they were known. And Gerry Sr. is here tonight, with his partner, Jill. Hello, Gerry and Jill! So, Little Gerry grew up on Wadland Crescent, in the east end of St. John's, joined after a few years by his sister, Lisa.

There was laughter at the baby pictures, and even louder laughter at the toddler photos.

Gerry was a pretty nerdy kid as evidenced by his choice of a best friend, Ed Riche. And that's the young Ed Riche, believe it or not. Also, as his classmate Mary Sexton informed us, Gerry was the only kid at Mary Queen of Peace who used Letraset for the title pages of all his class projects.

Loud laughter, followed by cheering and applause.

Growing up, Gerry spent lots of time with his Healey cousins from his mother's community of Blackhead. His first cousins Val, Vida, Bonnie, and Toni are here tonight. We call them the Healey cousins or the Ryan girls. Anyway, the Healeys are here in force tonight. Raise your hands, Healey cousins!

In the summers, Gerry's family would take trips to visit his father's family in Ontario where he was good pals with his first cousins, known in those days as the Huntley girls. And the Huntley girls are here tonight, two of them, Allison and Lorraine. Where are you, Huntley girls?

Gerry was always interested in drawing and cartoons. He and his friend Wallace Ryan did two issues of the magazine Zeitgeist *when they were in high school. And this is Gerry's cover that he spent endless hours drawing.* [loud applause]

At this point, two-year-old Ursula skipped over to Gerry and tried to climb on his lap. He smoothed her hair with one hand, holding his glass of wine in the other, and was rescued by Maggie, who carted her off.

Graduating from Gonzaga in 1979, Gerry started at MUN *at the tender age of seventeen. He was quickly captured by* The Muse *mafia* [cheering] *and met his good friends Tim Peckham and Dave Roe. Here is a cartoon of work he did at* The Muse, *"The Banana Republic."*

Gerry left MUN *before he finished his degree, drawn to the big lights of Ottawa and the lure of being president of Canadian University Press in 1983.* [hooting and clapping] *Here is a picture of him reporting on the Tory convention in, I guess, 1983.*

"Yes, 1983," Gerry called from the floor. "The one that Mulroney won." The audience groaned.

He may also have been drawn to Ottawa because his then-girlfriend Martha Muzychka was going to J-school *at Carleton.* [laughter]

Next thing you know, Gerry was back in St. John's, working for the Evening Telegram. *He did not really like working as a reporter, finding he had no talent for going to people's doors and inquiring how they felt about their personal disasters.*

"Just read that as no talent," called out Gerry.

There was loud laughter, caused by a photo of a very cute Gerry with long hair and a cigarette dangling from his lips, bending over a pool table, cue in hand.

So, he left for the greener pastures of Arts in formation— remember that?—where he worked with his then-girlfriend Joan Sullivan (these pool shots are him working, by the way) and made lots of funny cartoons. This one says, "The Despair of the '80s Meets the Irony of the '90s."

A second cartoon featured a Gerry-like figure slumped despairingly in front of a portable television, hands covering his face, saying, "God, they're all such assholes . . ." It was captioned, "My Very Last Editorial Cartoon."

Gerry and I got together in 1986, which resulted in the birth of Nicholas Robert McGee in August of 1987, when Gerry was only twenty-five. We did not become an actual couple until November 1988, and our first place together was the then NIFCO apartment, where we lived until we bought our house at 13 William Street, in June 1990. Our son Christopher William McGee was born in January 1991.

"*You* were born, Daddy!" Jack shouted.

Gerry was working at MUN Extension as a publications and information officer. When Extension was closed in 1991, Gerry was thankfully able to bump to what was then called Educational Technology, working as a graphic artist.

    By then we had started our own pattern of going to Ontario every second summer, visiting with my family and with Gerry's dad and his second family. Gerry became a great favourite with the McGees, doing hilarious Photoshop covers for our annual calendar.

The next minute featured sustained laughter and applause, as calendar spoofs of *The Sopranos, Lord of the Rings,* and *Twilight* were shown. The loudest laugh came for Occupy the McGees, our 2012 calendar.

> *I have family members who've come for this event tonight, my brother Jim and his wife, Debbie, and my sister Gail and brother Mark. Where are you, famloids? You're here somewhere.*
>
> *In the first decade of our life together, I made films and Gerry worked at* MUN. *He played poker every Thursday with his poker buddies. I invite any poker buddies who are here tonight to make some noise.* [deep-voiced shouts, clapping, and whistling]
>
> *He also did graphics and the website for his buddies at* The Great Eastern, *something that remains his passion till the current day.*

There were hoots of laughter at a Photoshop of the *Great Eastern* gang as outlaw gunslingers.

> *Gerry's sister, Lisa, became partners with Paul Pope, and they became parents too, of the delightful boys Simon and Alex. Hey, gang!*
>
> *We did our best to be good parents, which to us meant taking them to events at the* LSPU *Hall as often as possible, spending part of the Christmas holidays at John Koop's cabin in Tors Cove, and visiting Jane Robinson's cabin in Monkstown during our Newfoundland summers.*

In the second decade, I went to work at MUN in the same unit as Gerry, which was then called CAMS (the Centre for Academic and Media Services), as a video producer. People used to ask if it was a problem for us to work in the same unit, but aside from the car on the way to and from work, we didn't spend that much time together—at work. [long laughter]

In 2001, the summer before 9/11, we took our kids on a three-week trip to England and France. Gerry did a lot of travelling after that for work with trips to Uganda, Kenya, and Ukraine, as well as less exciting trips to Washington, Boston, San Jose, and San Francisco.

We got married in 2005.

A loud aw greeted a picture of Gerry and me on our wedding day, with applause for a photo of us kissing.

Gerry continued playing poker but less often, as most of the cards guys had families by then.

Gerry and Lisa's beloved mother, Ida, died in 2006. What a beauty.

"She was a great poker host," yelled a voice from the crowd.

Gerry was doing a lot of poster work for local theatre companies, c2c, Rabbittown, and Resource Centre for the Arts. Some of those posters are on the walls here tonight, and many of them are playing on the slide show. Thank you to Paul Pope and Benjy Kean and quite a few people at The Hall for helping to gather them.

I became a Buddhist in 2006, and a side of Gerry you would not guess, considering that he is a committed atheist [laughter], *is how supportive he has been of me and how much food he has made over the years for the Shambhala community and for Shambhala teachers.*

The kids grew up. Nick started university in 2005.

Chris started university in 2009.

Gerry became Lead Multimedia Specialist in what was then called DELT, Distance Education, Learning, and Technology.

In the current third decade, many exciting developments. Chris met and married the wonderful Maggie Burton, and we became the doting grandparents of Jack and Ursula McGee.

"That's me," Jack cried in ecstasy, as he saw his baby pictures, "that's me!" When the laughing died down, I resumed.

Jack and Ursula McGee, the prince and princess of Facebook.

Much laughter as Gerry's many selfies with the grandkids were shown.

Nick is now based in Toronto, where he is doing his doctorate in Chinese history, and he also has a wonderful partner, Caitlin Henry, who is here tonight as well. Hey, Caitlin!

In 2012, we bought our beloved house in Heart's Content, to which you're all invited.

"I've been to Heart's Content," Jack called out. "With you!"

We travelled to Cuba with my family, Tanzania with Nick, and went to Scotland by ourselves in 2015. [laughter]

I retired from DELTS (Distance Education, Learning, and Teaching Support!) in 2014. Sadly, we lost my mom, Janette McGee, in 2014, and my dad, Robert McGee, in 2015.

At the sight of the picture of my father, Jack called to me, "Grandma?"

"Yes, dear?" I replied from the stage.

"I know that guy. He's the trapdoor man, he played trapdoor with me."

"Yes, he did, that's your grandfather. I mean, your great-grandfather."

That brings us to 2016, which I refer to as the year of woe.

As if on cue, Ursula began crying loudly and uncontrollably. "Top people are working on it," I reassured the crowd. The next few remarks were to the background of tearful shrieks.

When Gerry was diagnosed with gliosarcoma in April of this year, we knew he would not have a long lifespan. Because they told us the stats—a 10 per cent chance of being alive in two years. Still, we decided to try our best, did all the treatments, and were able to attend Gerry's fave event, the Ottawa Jazz Festival.

Complete quiet in the room.

Unfortunately, we didn't get the breaks. A second tumour appeared. And before I move on, I don't know if you can read this slide—it's one of Gerry's cartoons. It says, "I'm sorry, I'm an ontologist. I can't cure your cancer, but I can prove you exist."

Ten seconds of heartfelt clapping, followed by a family picture of our Nova Scotia vacation.

We went on a holiday with our family in Nova Scotia for a week.

"Grandma, Grandpa!" Jack ran up to Gerry's wheelchair. "I went to Nova Scotia! Remember we went to the beach?"

"Yes, we went to the beach a lot!" I replied.

They had fun. And even Gerry had fun.

A picture of Gerry looking tiny in a gigantic red beach chair produced a huge burst of laughter.

Unfortunately, the tumour kept growing. A short second-course of radiation has slowed it down. But we were advised to make our plans for the end. (That's our cat, Freya.)

With Gerry being the supreme atheist, a memorial party was planned instead of a funeral service. In the past month, we decided to have that party now, while Gerry is still with us. And so here we are.

Long, loud, sustained applause, shouting, hooting.

And so, what can I say to end this? I'm sure each one of you is more than aware how difficult this is for us. But as Marty Sexton said, it's the price of admission. And we've had a very fortunate life, with all the things one could hope for in a life. And you have each been a part of that life, in ways large and small, and we thank you so much for that, and for being here with us tonight.

During the lengthy applause that followed, I stepped off the stage and hugged Lisa as she rose from her chair and made way for me. Gerry took my hand and kissed it, and I turned his wheelchair so we could watch the next speakers. We were on full display, next to the stage. I sat close beside him, my arm on his shoulders, as Nick stood at the podium.

For those of you who don't know me, I'm Gerry's son Nick. Although I'm not quite as cute as I was in those baby photos, I'm not entirely without my charms. Thanks so much for singing back there, I was very moved.

You've heard some great things about Dad as a husband and a friend and an artist, but I thought that I'd say something about Gerry as a father, since there are only two of us around who can speak to the experience of being his children—as far as I know.

Immense laughter. Gerry shrugged, raising his eyebrows and making a "who knows?" gesture with his hands. We grinned at each other.

The incredible creativity you can see on the walls here, this is something that Dad used to add colour to the lives of his kids. In our family archive, we have these fantastic comics that Dad did with Chris and me when we were kids, when we were on family vacation, in which Chris and I would come up with a fantastical story, and Dad would draw it panel by panel, while we excitedly dictated what would happen next.

Gerry removed his glasses and began to wipe his eyes with a finger.

Dad is a fantastic cook, and virtually every day of my life when I lived at home, he would prepare a family dinner for us all, even when time or money was short, and I genuinely believe that sitting down all together as a family every night to eat was an important part of my development as a person.

This is just one of the ways I think Dad tried to pass on to his kids the qualities of generosity and a love of creativity. I think that Chris and I have inherited a lot from my dad, and I don't just mean male-pattern baldness. [laughter] *It's coming for you too, Chris.* [laughter]

I think Dad instilled in us a profound intellectual curiosity as well, a real love of learning. In the days well before the invention of Wikipedia, Dad's friends would actually call him to ask him trivia questions when they were stumped, because there was a good chance he would know the answer. As a child I used to say that I wanted to grow up to know as much stuff as my dad. At almost thirty, I don't know if I can say that I've succeeded, but at least I've learned enough to be able to say when he's full of it. [loud laughter] *Just kidding!*

Humour is another one of Dad's great qualities.

The audience burst into clapping and hooting, various shouts of "yeah!" ringing out.

And I can tell you we were steeped in it as children. Dad has always had a very sharp wit and a keen observational sense of humour, which can be a little bit difficult to render in anecdote. But as you know, in recent years Dad has taken to social media as a platform for his comedy and, among other things, has amassed quite a following. So, I thought I'd just use a few of those as an illustration of his sense of humour.

I dug back into the ether of Dad's first tweet, November 2, 2011. Here goes. "Hoping this first tweet is a good one. Oh shit . . ."

The audience roared. I did too. Gerry removed his glasses, put them back on, and took a steadying sip from his wine glass.

Here's one of my Twitter favourites, a film parody, from July 2013. It's in four parts.

Mercantile Park: Wealthy industrialist modeled on Zita Cobb uses DNA from pork barrels to recreate 19th century NL fishing village…

…complete with planters, merchants, and priests. A massive tourist attraction is established on Fogo Island with these beings…

…but they run amok, killing tourists and reverting to a state of harsh and primitive social relations common to their period.

Fogo is sealed off to the outside world. Movie ends on eerie bellowing sound, with accordions, echoing over water. Hashtag, GreenlightThis

Sustained laughter and applause. Ursula climbed on to my lap, her little yellow boots swinging against my legs. I kissed her hair.

Finally, something I know that both Chris and I have learned from you, Dad, is the importance of love and respect for strong, caring, capable, feminist women, and I'd like to take a moment before I step down to thank Mom for making this event possible, for looking out for Dad and for me and all of us at this point in our lives.

Through the clapping that followed, Ursula jumped down, tugging at my hand with all her might, trying to get me to follow her. When that failed, she took Gerry's hand, pulling at him like a horse with a cart. Her mother intervened and carried her away, as Nick finished speaking.

I love you, Dad.

"I love *you*, Uncle Nick," Jack called out.
    "I love you, too, Jack," Nick responded.

I've been very lucky to have you as a father and as a friend for the past thirty years, and I consider myself privileged to spend this chapter of your life with you.

Long, long applause. Gerry wiped his eyes and I hugged him to me as Nick stepped down from the stage. Next came Chris, tall and handsome, juggling microphone and notebook. Gerry put his wine glass between his legs.

First, I'd like to say thank you to Nick and thank you to Mom for speaking so eloquently to Dad's life, and thanks for putting this whole thing together.

Gerry had tears running down his face as he joined in the applause.

Thanks to all of you for coming. This is so wonderful and moving to see all of you here.

Gerry began exhaling, trying to gain composure. I rubbed his shoulders. He took off his glasses and wiped his eyes. Chris continued.

Since becoming a parent myself, I felt a deeper appreciation of what it means to be a parent—after having kids, it's only then that you realize how much sheer hard work and dedication and love that your parents had to put into your life to make you survive. [laughter] *I feel a lot of affinity for Dad as a fellow person who came into parenthood probably earlier than they were expecting.* [laughter] *I feel that we're kindred spirits in that regard.* [loud laughter]

Ursula leaned on the stage, holding her arms up to Chris, but when he responded with only "Hey, baby," she ran behind Gerry and me, crowing happily.

Dad has been a wonderful role model for me, in terms of being a parent and showing up and putting in the work every single day. It's really wonderful that you did that for Nick and me, and we really appreciate that.

    Boy. There's a lot of people here. [laughter] *Thank you for being a wonderful grandfather to my two children. You've always been patient and kind and loving to them, and they absolutely love you as much as I do. So, thank you. I'm extremely grateful you were able to be a part of their lives.*

Gerry looked to the ceiling, taking deep breaths. I passed him a tissue.

Probably the biggest effect that Dad has had on my life is that he passed on to me his love of music. It's probably had the most profound effect on my life and my personal aesthetics. His love of music is fearless and omnivorous. He's probably the biggest music enthusiast that I know, and it's that spirit of adventure

that I aspire to carry on in my own music making and my
listening.

Gerry took off his glasses and wiped his eyes with the tissue.

We're going to establish a scholarship, or a bursary—it will be
called The Gerry Porter Award for Creative Improvised Music.

During the explosion of hooting and clapping that followed, Ursula draped herself on the side of Gerry's wheelchair. He put his arm around her and rubbed her back as she gazed up at him. Then she moved away and joined in the clapping.

Further details to follow, but basically it will be a cash award,
administered by me and Mack Furlong. Contact Mom if you're
interested in learning more about this.
    Thank you to all of you for coming. It really means the
world to us. And I want to say thank you to Dad, for being who
you are. Thank you for being in our lives. We all really love you.

"Yeah, I love you, Grandpa!" Jack shouted.
    There was laughter and clapping as Chris left the stage and kissed his father on the top of his head.
    Then it was Ed's turn.

I have been playing with Gerry Porter since 1967. [laughter]
The houses we grew up in backed on one another. A tall fence
separated our yards. Our parents didn't want us climbing over
the fence, but we couldn't be stopped, so they cut a gate in the
thing, like something for pets.

Gerry was wiping his eyes. Jack and Ursula were crouched behind my chair, poking me. I played along, feigning indignation to their great amusement, while keeping one hand on Gerry's shoulder and listening to Ed.

Since we left those neighbouring suburban houses, Gerry and I have gone on to share four separate addresses.

So I know this man well and could tell you much about his character: creative force; super dad and grandfather; the best big brother; critical thinker; a brilliant graphic artist with the old-school newspaper editor's insistence on clarity; hilarious cartoonist; beloved boss; and of course, the love of Debbie's life. All that. But what most marks this man is his generosity, his tirelessly giving so freely of his time, his wisdom, and his spirit. In a world with so many takers and users, Gerry is one of the makers and givers. [loud applause]

Gerry was mopping his eyes constantly now. I rubbed his shoulders. I was also laughing at the jokes.

Now, lest you think I'm describing some paragon [laughter]*, I have seen Gerry fume and stomp and storm. You see, because of his core spirit of giving and sharing, there is something pink in his politics, and he cannot abide greed. Seeing avarice, reading about it—up goes Ger. It's something to witness. I love it. Twitter loves it.* [laughter]

Gerry and I are part of a poker game that has been going on for thirty years. To the younger players it's known as the-old-guys-screaming-at-one-another game. [laughter] *Some of our game's players are that fond of Ger that they flew down to attend this event tonight—Luke Major, Andrew Younghusband, Steve Cochrane, Dave Roe.* [long applause]

Ursula was once again balancing on the wheelchair. Her mother tried to lure her away, but instead Ursula climbed on the stage, sitting just out of reach.

That poker game isn't about the gambling—the small stakes have never really changed. It's about the talk, the scurrilous, bawdy talk, and the laughter. Jaysus Murphy, the hours and hours of laughter from around that table. I've genuinely worried that Dave Roe or Johnny Housser were about to expire from laughter. I have, on many occasions, witnessed Gerry, at that game, crying from laughter.

We around that table have gotten more than our fair share of Gerry's quick wit. And we at that game say of the best sort of conduct, the finest examples of humanity, of smarts and a large heart, we say, "Good man! Top man!" And he is. A toast, please, to our great, great friend, that I love, Gerry Porter!

Gerry put his arm around my shoulders, and I held his hand. Everyone with a glass raised it to Gerry. Lengthy applause and hooting followed.

Then came the official photo shoot, with the photographer we had hired taking group shots of the family. There are many photos of Gerry and me from that night, exchanging looks, laughing, and hugging one another.

A second service of the same appetizers was set out and, again, quickly devoured. There was laughter, tears, many pictures taken, and a special presentation to Gerry from "the cards guys." It was uncanny to see so many people from the different walks of our lives, all gathered in one room. Old neighbours, family from both near and far, our closest friends, work friends, arts community friends, Shambhala friends, and even our kids' friends. I flitted about the room chatting, receiving hugs, and urging people to sign the guestbook. Every time someone asked me, "How are you?" I responded with an enthusiastic, "Fantastic!" Because the event was everything we had hoped it would be, and I was so happy for Gerry.

Toward the end of the night, Gerry was receiving a long line of people who wanted to speak to him in person. I knew he must be exhausted, but he refused to take a break, and there was no way I was going to impose my will in that environment. Nick and I exchanged worried glances, but it was Gerry's last party, and he could do what he wanted.

———

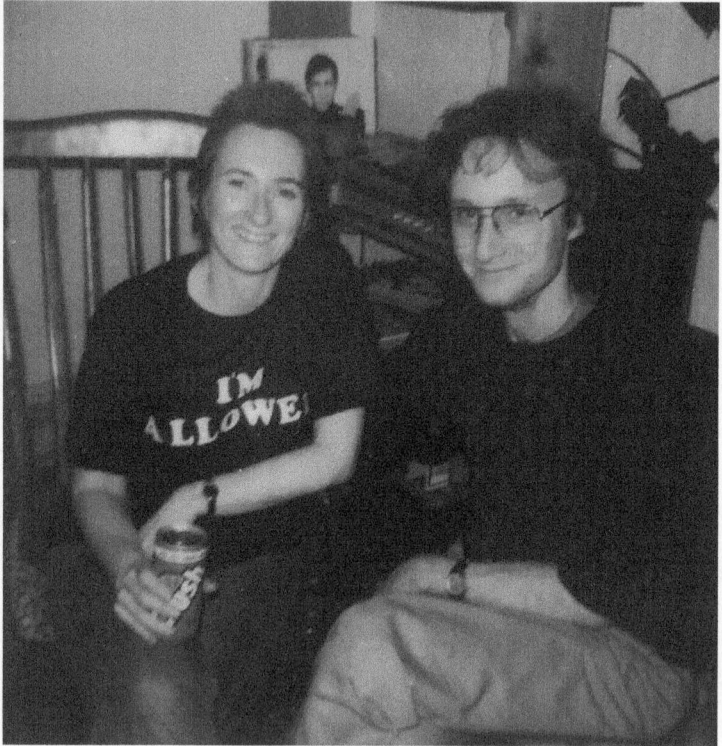

EIGHT

After the Terms of Union in November 1988, Gerry and I lived together for twenty-eight years, years that for the most part were far less dramatic than our rocky beginning.

I met his mother, he met my parents and siblings, and on one of those trips to Ottawa, Gerry and his father reconciled.

There was a happy ending to the saga of my film project. Released in 1989 under the name *Multiple Choice*, it was nominated for a Genie Award. In March 1990, Gerry and I flew to Toronto for the ceremony, leaving Nick behind with our sitter. It was our first holiday alone together, something not to be repeated for twenty-five years.

Nick would soon be three years old, we were buying a house, and it felt like the right time to grow our family. In February of 1990, we decided to try for a second child. As soon as we stopped using birth control, I was hired by the Provincial Advisory Council on the Status of Women to direct three ads and a short film for *Imagine That!*, a campaign designed to interest young women in non-traditional jobs. I was also working on *Toward Intimacy*, a documentary on women, disability, and sexuality, with Studio D, the women's studio at the National Film Board of Canada. Maybe we should put off getting pregnant? But it was too late. The baby was due in January 1991. I accepted the contracts anyway.

Gerry admitted to being somewhat impressed that our bodies worked so efficiently. "Me too," I said, "from a Darwinian perspective, at least."

We moved into our new house on William Street during the *Imagine That!* shoot. It was only a few blocks from the NIFCO apartment, in Georgestown. It had three bedrooms and a backyard and would be perfect for raising two children. I was now four months pregnant, and Gerry had to paint the interior by himself. He was still working at MUN Extension and finishing his degree, one course a semester.

Since I was thirty-seven years old, this was considered a geriatric pregnancy. I had an amniocentesis, a procedure where the fluid surrounding the baby is analyzed for possible birth defects. The obstetrician called with the results when I was in editing at NIFCO. I remember stretching the phone cord out into the hallway and time being suspended while I waited to hear if the baby was genetically sound. Yes!

"Do you want to know the gender?"

"Yes, please."

"It's a boy."

"Oh," I said, "I was really hoping for a girl."

The obstetrician scolded me. "You have a healthy baby. That's all that matters!"

I've felt guilty ever since.

On August 19, 1990, we threw a big housewarming party for Nick's third birthday. With our new house and a new baby on the way, we felt pleased to demonstrate to our friends and family that our relationship was on solid ground.

When fall arrived, Gerry's union was on strike. He spent his days on the picket line, while I was shooting the St. John's section of *Toward Intimacy*. The strike ended and the film shoot finished up in December. We were ready for our first Christmas in our new house, with a very excited Nicholas. I was hugely pregnant, having gained forty pounds. Over the holidays we watched *Total Recall* with Arnold Schwarzenegger. It became one of our Christmas movies from then on, along with *A Christmas Carol* and *Scrooged*.

I was happy that Gerry would be present for the birth of his second son. It would be like wiping the slate clean. But as the due date approached, I developed an infection. It was diagnosed as herpes, and I was told a normal delivery would mean risking blindness and mental disability for the baby.

Christopher William McGee was born by Caesarean section on January 5, 1991, in an operating room packed with residents, warm blankets, tents, and an epidural. Gerry held my hand throughout. Our birthing picture is Gerry in blue scrubs, shower cap, and face mask, cuddling newborn Chris, who is staring up at him. I'm still on the operating table, peeking out around them, smiling.

Gerry loved tending the baby. Baths, diapering, endless soothing—everything he had missed the first time round. A few months after Chris was born, Memorial University decided to close MUN Extension, and Gerry's job abruptly ended.

"I talked to the union. I feel kind of bad, but I've got enough seniority to bump somebody over at Ed Tech."

And so began his career as a graphic artist at Memorial University. He took a cut in pay, but under the circumstances, we were relieved he had a job at all.

When Chris was six months old, I went across Canada on a ten-day film shoot for *Toward Intimacy*. I dithered on whether to take the baby with me, as I was still breast-feeding. In the end, I decided Chris would be safer at home. Gerry took the time off. Our babysitter came every day, and Gerry made a deck in our fledgling backyard. In July of 1992, I shot a film on youth and HIV / AIDS for the Atlantic NFB, *Thinking Positive*. Each film had to be edited, had to be launched, had to be promoted. Without the internet, everything was organized by phone or through the postal system and by physically travelling to the meeting or the event.

How many times did Gerry look after the kids over those first ten years, while I went to film festivals, film conferences, film screenings, and film shoots in and out of the province? I went to Toronto, Halifax, Montreal, Vancouver, Victoria, Winnipeg, Yorkton, Edmonton, Munich, Cannes, London, New York, and Paris and Los Angeles twice each. I have no recollection of him ever complaining or making me feel guilty for being away and the extra work it caused him. He was always supportive of my career, while caring for gerbils and dogs and cooking supper for fussy children. In fact, he developed great skill as a cook, eventually taking over supper duties completely. His sausage spaghetti sauce was and still is a family favourite at Porter-McGee gatherings. Gerry was also heavily involved with *The Great Eastern* during this period, from 1994 to 1999.

In 1996, three film projects of mine received funding. One I had to give up, but the other two went into production: *The Elf*, a short drama for Global TV, and *Untidy Package*, an NFB documentary on women and the cod moratorium. As is the nature of the business, each project was fraught with difficult challenges, and by the time 1998 rolled around, I was depressed and anxious, and unsure of my future.

I didn't feel able to handle the stresses and unpredictability of freelance life anymore. Nick was eleven and Chris was seven, and both were in school in the day. When a job opened at Memorial University, in the same department where Gerry was now head of graphic services, I decided to apply.

In October 1998, I went to work as a producer-director in the video section of the Centre for Academic and Media Services, which soon had a name change to Distance Education and Learning Technology. The workload was varied, from closed-circuit, live psychology lectures, videos for distance education courses, promotional videos for various academic departments, and occasionally, meatier projects such as documentaries and educational dramas.

It was a completely different work environment from my career as an independent filmmaker. There was much less travel. There was no hiring of crew or renting equipment on a project-by-project basis. The camera operators and the editor were on staff, and the necessary equipment was already on hand. We even had our own cars and trucks. I didn't have to raise any money, just stay within my budget. And I got paid every two weeks! Although it was less glamorous and had less status than my work as an independent filmmaker, it was the perfect job for me. I was grateful for the stability and the security. Gerry and I drove to and from work together for the next fifteen years.

———

Like all couples, over the years our relationship went through ups and downs. After we got back together in 1988, we were lovebirds for the first few years, holding hands when out in the pubs, making love most nights. The passion quotient went down once we had both a baby and a three-year-old and very few full nights of sleep.

One night in 1991, we were folding baby laundry on the bed, and Gerry told me that an old girlfriend had a weekly gig reviewing films. She received free passes and had asked if he wanted to go with her.

"What do you think?" he asked. I glanced over at Chris, sleeping in his crib a few feet away.

"What do I think about you going to the movies with a woman who broke your heart and is just out of a relationship? While I stay home with two kids?" I placed a striped sleeper on the pile. "Go ahead if you want, but you probably won't be living here."

He didn't even seem surprised. "Okay, no problem. I don't have to go."

Was my reaction too strong? I don't know which of my various indoctrinations were operating, but I couldn't even begin to handle the stress of wondering if they would have an affair. I needed to know he was with me, and only me.

I hope Gerry was faithful to me during our time together, but I know I was faithful to him, even if I did sometimes show dreadful judgment in flirting and drinking with men at festivals and workplaces. But as the decades rolled on, it was hard to remember that our relationship was once the talk of the town. We were an established couple, with two kids, two dogs, two cats, and two jobs.

Not that we didn't have problems over the twenty-eight years. Money was a stressor in the first decade. It's expensive to have two children, and mortgage rates were high in the 1990s. I made more than Gerry did, both as a freelancer and as a producer-director, but he had the skills to make extra money through freelance work or teaching night courses. Sometimes it seemed he was always at work. It took several years for us to put our money in a joint account and use it for all our expenses. That was a big step in affirming our intention to stay together, maybe even more than having a second child!

We had always been good at making joint decisions on the house and the kids. We had similar design tastes and could easily agree on which sofa to purchase, what bedsheets we liked, the colours for the walls. But somehow, somewhere in 1999, we stopped getting along. Something as simple as how to wash lettuce or where to put the raked leaves could lead to an argument. My feminism won out over my 1950s childhood, and it seemed wrong not to respond when I felt he was demeaning me. I was increasingly unhappy, and our rides to and from work were silently tense.

In August 1999 we took the kids on a ten-day camping trip across Newfoundland. This was a big concession on Gerry's part, as he hated camping, but hotels were too expensive. We were headed for the Viking encampment at L'Anse aux Meadows on the Great Northern Peninsula. We rented a tent trailer, to avoid sleeping on the ground. Gerry backed it into a tree our first night out, which didn't help his mood. The kids, twelve and eight, seemed to have fun, but from choosing the camping spot to erecting the dining tent, there's plenty to argue about on a trip like this, and we bickered from our first night in Terra Nova to Nick's twelfth birthday in Grand Falls-Windsor, from Shallow Bay in Gros Morne to L'Anse aux Meadows, and all the way home to St. John's.

By fall 1999, I was feeling we would have to separate. Listening to *Morningside* in the car on my way back to MUN one morning, I heard an interview with a woman who had just written a book on divorce. I pulled into a parking lot to listen. When asked what advice she would give to persons contemplating such a move, she replied, "Divorce is an absolute last resort. It is one of the worst life events you will ever experience, and the pain lasts for years. Make sure you have tried everything else first."

Her sincerity impressed me. Although we weren't married, there were the children to consider. Many of their school friends' parents' marriages had ended. We had previously joked that they didn't have to worry, we'd already done that. But now Gerry and I were scoring points for various things we did for the family ("Well, *I* went shopping!" "Yeah, well *I* cleaned the whole house *and* did the laundry!"), and I was not wanting to give any ground to him. Still, in the spirit of trying everything first, I suggested we needed to talk.

That night, after the kids had gone to bed, we faced each other in the kitchen. Standing in front of our Claude Monet wall calendar, I asked why he was always so rude to me.

"You have no respect for me," he replied. "You think I'm a loser, and a lousy father."

"I think no such thing! I think you are very hard-working and talented and a great father! I just can't stand the way you treat me."

Once we realized that neither of us hated the other, we began to get along again. It was as simple as that. Why is communicating so hard? It's astounding that we could have separated, based on faulty assumptions about what the other was thinking and feeling. I'm so grateful to the CBC.

Better communication wasn't the only thing that helped us get along. In 1999, I made *Out of the Dark*, a video on youth and depression, for the Newfoundland division of the Canadian Mental Health Association. Thank goodness the project was assigned to me, because it changed my life. Not only did I learn enough about depression that I got counselling and medication, but my association with the executive director of the CMHA turned into a deep friendship that led me to Shambhala Buddhism in 2000.

With the depression lifted, the glass of my life went from half-empty to half-full. The unread books on my shelf were no longer a reproach to me, a mark of my failure. Instead they were an exciting opportunity, full of promise. My energy increased, and I became more patient, due also to the Buddhist teachings I was studying. All this had a healthy impact on our relationship.

Gerry made an effort, too. He was hilarious, but he could also be a fusspot. As he learned to hold back on his complaints, and I learned to not take his testiness personally, daily life became far less stressful. We divided up the housework in a way that fit our needs: Gerry did the cooking, the car, and the garbage; I did the laundry and the garden. We shared the shopping, bathrooms, vacuuming, dog walking, and taking the children to their many activities. We were able to relax and enjoy the things that we liked about each other—humour, curiousity, creativity. Our close ties with his family in St. John's and my family in Ontario created another strong bond.

Plus, our roles changed. After 2001, Gerry began to travel nationally and internationally for work, and I was the person who stayed home with the kids. I gained a new appreciation for how much time it takes to do all the driving, care for the kids and animals, and manage the house on your own—plus work full-time.

In 2005, I took six months off, coping with a return of depression brought on by an increasingly chaotic situation at work. Since we were in the same department, Gerry knew all about the problems I faced and was supportive, encouraging me to do what I needed to regain strength and stamina. He was also freelancing as a graphic artist, making posters for local theatre companies.

But there were more changes afoot. From a 2005 letter to a friend:

> *Gerry's mother, who lives on her own, has Alzheimer's, and over the past year it has progressed pretty rapidly. She comes to our house or Lisa's house every night for supper and has a part-time home care worker during the days when she's not at daycare. We are now beginning the application process to get her into a seniors' home, as she is declining to the point where we don't feel she is safe at night anymore.*

In July of 2005, Mrs. Porter entered a care home. Clearing her house as we prepared to sell it, I found boxes of Gerry's old drawings and newspaper clippings of articles he had written while working at the *Evening Telegram* in the 1980s. They all ended up under our bed.

We spent several weeks in Ontario that summer of 2005, and when we returned home, Gerry and I decided to get married. We joked it was the only way to lure my parents to Newfoundland. I had never been a believer in marriage, but now it seemed like a good idea. The kids were almost grown, eighteen and fourteen, so it wasn't for their benefit, although they seemed quite pleased, but it would be good for pension-sharing, wills, and the financial concerns of later life. And also, maybe, the security of a public commitment to one another, which both of us were ready to make.

We decided to invite only immediate relatives, as too many feelings might be hurt if we chose friends, and we couldn't afford to ask all of them. On Thanksgiving weekend of 2005, my parents, my three sisters, and my older brother and his wife came to witness our wedding, joined by Lisa, Paul, and their children, Simon and Alex, as well as Gerry's father.

We were married by a Justice of the Peace in a cozy two-room restaurant on Cookstown Road that specialized in catering private events. My sisters and I had come by earlier in the day and decorated the front room as a wedding chapel, setting out vases of sunflowers, chairs for twelve guests, and placing a white room divider as a backdrop at the front, where the vows would take place. Gerry and I had chosen white calla lilies as our wedding flower, with Gerry, Chris, Nick, and our fathers wearing boutonnieres, my mother a corsage, while I carried a calla lily bouquet.

Gerry and I made our entrance from the back room, walking arm-in-arm to the strains of the wedding march from *Lieutenant Kijé* by Prokofiev. I was wearing a dark-brown, full-length wool skirt, a cream silk blouse, and a dark brown silk scarf with gold embroidery. Gerry had on a black suit with a burgundy shirt and tie. We joined the Justice of the Peace (resplendent in full black robes, with two dashing red stripes and a dazzling white lawyer's band) and our sons (wearing suits and ties) in front of the white divider.

In front of our family, we faced each other holding hands. Our two sons, both about six feet tall, stood with us: Nick behind Gerry and Chris behind me. We had considered writing our own vows, but both of us felt the words of the civil ceremony were complete. The judge had us each repeat the wedding vow. Gerry went first.

"I call upon all persons present to witness that I, Gerry, do take you, Debra, to be my lawful wedded wife, to have and to hold from this day forward, for better, for worse, for richer, for poorer, in sickness and in health, to love and to cherish, and I pledge to you my faithful love."

I repeated the vow back to Gerry, and we exchanged rings. The judge asked us to hold hands and stand side by side, facing our family. Together, we repeated after him, "This is my beloved, and this is my friend." We beamed at each other. I saw both of my parents wipe their eyes.

The judge knew we had two sons but somehow hadn't grasped they were the two young giants beside us. After pronouncing us married, he said, "Now I'd like to invite your sons to come up and join their parents." He beckoned to our bewildered nephews, twelve-year-old Simon and seven-year-old Alex, sitting in the back next to Lisa and Paul. There was momentary confusion, followed by much laughter, as we introduced the Justice to Nick and Chris.

The chairs were pushed to the side of the room, and as our wedding song, "Harvest Moon" by Neil Young, played on the speakers, Gerry and I began waltzing. Soon everyone joined in. After signing the register and posing for photos, we moved to the next room where three banquet tables were set up in a semicircle for a mad swirl of toasts, appetizers, roast pork loin with braised Savoy cabbage, bittersweet chocolate torte, and speeches.

The next day, we held a reception at our home for friends and family. The weather was fair, and our guests crowded in the kitchen, living room, and under a canopy tent in the backyard, drinking wine and munching a layered wedding cake made by my good friend Jane Robinson. How fortunate we were to have so much love in our life! I still wear my wedding ring, but on my right hand.

We would have liked to go for a honeymoon, especially to New York City, but since I was still off work, it was financially out of the question. We'd go another time.

―――

On February 14, 2006, Gerry's mother died suddenly. Gerry and Lisa were present, thank goodness. I flew home from rural Nova Scotia, where I was attending a Shambhala retreat. It was our first personal experience of the comfort friends, family, and community can bring at a time of loss, and from then on it affected my own outlook on the importance of attending wakes. Go if you can. You will never regret going, but you might regret not going. A day after the funeral, I asked Gerry if he minded if I returned to the retreat.

"Can you stay one more day?" he said. I was touched. It wasn't common for Gerry to express emotional needs, and I was happy he had asked.

At our local retreat in April of that year, I formally became a Buddhist by taking the refuge vow, in which one takes refuge in the Buddha, the dharma, and the sangha. What I like about Buddhism is that Buddha is not a god, and the view of human nature is one of fundamental goodness. This does not mean we don't get confused and make mistakes! But the confusion is viewed like clouds—underneath, the sun is brilliantly clear, and this is true of everyone, no matter what they've done. This appeals to me so much more than the doctrine of original sin.

Gerry and Chris came to witness the ceremony. Gerry was always supportive of my Buddhist path and never questioned the money I spent attending Shambhala programs in St. John's or around the world, nor the immense amount of time I put in volunteering with the local group. As the years went on, we would frequently host visiting teachers, and Gerry became a great favourite, both for his wit and his French Onion Chicken with *Gruyère*.

―――

On November 13, 2008, I picked up Chris from his music lesson, dropped him at home, and walked over to Holy Heart High School, where I was meeting Gerry for a concert. There was an ambulance parked outside. I saw a crying girl nearby, being comforted by someone I knew from the film world. They were talking to a police officer. When I got into the auditorium, I couldn't find Gerry anywhere. I saw mutual acquaintances; nobody had seen him. I walked outside and regarded the ambulance with some suspicion. I called Chris to see if his dad had returned to the house. No.

I checked the auditorium again, this time saying to a seated friend, "I'm beginning to worry he could be in the ambulance."

"Don't be silly," she said. "He's just late."

The concert began. I went back to the lobby. The ambulance had gone. My phone rang.

"Hello, Debbie. This is Ann Marie Vaughan." The director of our unit at MUN, the big boss. "Do you know where Gerry is?"

"I'm beginning to think he is in an ambulance that just left," I said.

"Yes. He is. I just got a phone call from Doreen Neville [her big boss]. Gerry was hit by a car at the crosswalk in front of Holy Heart, and she was first on the scene. She recognized Gerry and called me, figuring I would know how to get hold of you. I called your house, and your son gave me your cell number."

This was St. John's. A town so small you can see someone get hit by a car and realize you not only know them, but you also know who they work for. And not only that, I was also beginning to realize I probably knew the people who had hit him.

First, I called Chris, who was by then understandably upset by all the phone calls regarding his dad's whereabouts. We went to the hospital together, receiving an official notification from the emergency department as we drove there.

When we got to the hospital, Doreen Neville was waiting for us. She wanted to explain in person what she had witnessed, knowing I would have many questions. Apparently, Gerry had gone over the hood, hit the road, and passed out briefly. Doreen had been a nurse before she became a university administrator, and so she used her best techniques to assess his level of consciousness while waiting for the ambulance. She reported he didn't know what had happened to him, but he did know his name.

I thanked her profusely, and we were led off to find Gerry, who was lying on a table in a trauma room. His clothes were torn, his face was scratched and bloody, there was a giant lump on his forehead, and one of his eyes was swollen shut. But apart from the loss of his top front teeth, it seemed no serious damage had been done. They wanted to send him home, and he wanted to go.

Gerry was off work for two weeks recovering from the bruises and cuts and general pain. I was so grateful I hadn't lost him and that the damage was minimal. There were psychological scars for both of us, though, being reminded so forcefully that life is precious and can end without warning. We had always known this intellectually and always kissed or at least said goodbye before leaving the house. That way, if something bad happened to the other person while separated, you would never have to regret your last words to them. Now we doubled down on that, even if it meant going upstairs or into the backyard to find each other before leaving.

But our jangled nerves still needed soothing. We still hadn't gone to New York City, but we decided what we needed most was to go somewhere warm and lie around on a beach, a holiday that had never appealed to us before. We joined my family for a week in Cuba in March of 2010.

After Gerry was diagnosed, I asked the oncologist if the concussion from the accident could have contributed to his cancer developing. He said, "I'll note it in his file. It would take a large research study to prove any correlation. But you never know."

On a positive note, the periodontist refused to replace Gerry's front teeth with implants if he was a cigarette smoker. So after almost thirty years of sometimes heavy smoking, Gerry quit with the aid of a smoking cessation program offered by our workplace.

In the years after the car accident, many things changed.

In 2009, Chris entered music school at Memorial University, studying saxophone. There he met Maggie, a violinist. Early in 2011, they informed us they were expecting a baby.

Although we received the news calmly, privately we were aghast. "Even if they were engineers," I moaned, "but musicians..."

They were both nineteen, in second year music school, and currently living at our house. But by the time the baby was due, they had borrowed a car from her grandparents, rented a house five minutes away from us, and finished another two semesters toward their degrees.

Jack Robert McGee was born on December 8, 2011, bringing delight and a new kind of love into our life.

Email to a friend:

Thursday, December 8, 2011

Yes, I think being a grandparent is going to be just fine. The kids can't believe how much the baby eats and how often he poops! I have to hide my chuckle. Gerry was cooking supper for them most nights before the baby arrived, and he will keep doing that, so we see them every day, which is nice. I'm delighted that they don't live with us though. Better for them and for us. But we have no children at home for Christmas for the first time in 24 years—we feel like orphans!

Both Maggie and Chris graduated with their cohort in spring of 2013. Adorable toddler Jack figures prominently in the graduation photos, peeking out between the black robes and tasselled hats. Chris and Maggie planned to get married in Brigus in August of 2013, and Gerry and I spent our winter weekends driving up to Heart's Content, where we had bought a small home on the road to the lighthouse. We wanted it to be ready to house wedding guests and spent enjoyable hours cleaning and decorating. My father had been enthusiastically rallying my siblings and their spouses to attend the wedding, and in the end, ten of them did come—but Mom and Dad cancelled at the last minute. Ostensibly, this was because Mom needed more time to recover from a knee replacement operation. But after the wedding, Dad revealed the real reason was that Mom's cancer had returned, for the third time.

I was in Ottawa in January 2014 when my mother was told her prognosis was terminal. With treatment, she might live till the fall. Mom decided she did not want to try chemotherapy. At best, it would give her only a little more time, and at worst, make her last months deeply unpleasant. I stayed in Ottawa for six weeks, relishing the time I spent with her.

In April 2014, shortly after I returned home, I retired from the university. Gerry was not certain when he would join me. He would turn fifty-five in three years, at which point he would be eligible to retire with a full pension, but he liked working. I did not try to convince him. I figured that three years of him going to work while I travelled, hung out at Heart's Content, and played with the grandchildren (Maggie was expecting another baby) would do more to change his mind about retirement than any debate could accomplish.

In May I received a text from my sister Gail, saying that Mom was doing poorly and I should come to Ottawa as soon as possible. Mom had been fine a week earlier when I spoke to her on Mother's Day. But within that week, she had stopped eating and drinking as a result of an esophageal stent we all thought was going to prolong and improve her life.

Gail was living with my parents now, and my sisters Robin and Jan and I came as soon as we could. We spelled each other off, visiting with Mom, getting up in the night, and keeping Dad in check.

From my journal:

May 23, 2014
The hospital bed arrived in the morning. It took two of us holding her on either side to walk her very slowly and carefully the 20 feet or so from one bed to another. She was astoundingly weak. Still cheerful though!

June 1, 2014
Mom seemed excessively quiet, and we felt this could be it. We called the brothers to come over. There were approximately ten of us, taking turns sitting beside her, taking our leave. Suddenly, she perked up, astounding us. "What are you all doing here?" she said. "I'm not going yet. I want to watch Game of Thrones *tonight."*

Afterwards, we joked, calling it a rehearsal. Most of us stayed to watch GoT with her. She slept through the episode, waking up at one point to say, "I know how it ends, anyway."

June 2, 2014
The sisters were out on the deck, putting a big flank steak on the barbeque. I went back to sit beside Mom. Dad was there too,

very depressed, slumped in the chair. I felt Mom's breathing was becoming irregular. Breathe in, breathe out. Breathe in, breathe out. Then a longer period before the next inhalation. After some time, Mom suddenly sat up, her eyes wide open. Then they rolled toward the ceiling, showing her whites in a rather frightening way. I pointed this out to Dad, but he just shrugged his shoulders.

I realized that if something was happening, it was up to me to let the sisters know. It was around 6:15 p.m. I went out to the deck and said, "Mom opened her eyes and rolled them and her breathing is funny." No one understood me. I said, "I think you'd better come."

They trailed after me, Gail telling Robin that it was her turn to learn how to give injections. I was doubtful there would be any more injections, but I'd been wrong before.

Mom's breathing was more and more irregular. We took turns holding her hands, patting her, murmuring our final words to her.

Death itself seemed very gentle. She breathed out and didn't inhale. There was no gasping. After a long time had passed and she didn't breathe, we all acknowledged she was gone. She was so still. Her skin had a yellowish hue. She just did not look alive. After some moments we left Dad with her and shut the door, while we phoned the brothers. It was about 6:45. They all said they would come immediately. I texted Gerry and the boys. Mom has died.

Mom had not wanted a church funeral, and Dad was so grief-stricken he did not want any kind of memorial service. Gerry was not happy about this. He loved my mom, and he wanted to come to Ottawa and pay his respects. I would have liked him there, too. The immediate family did manage a few words of remembrance in the living room, led by my Aunt Pat, Dad's sister, with Dad sitting morosely on the couch.

A few months later, our second grandchild, Ursula Ivy McGee, was born on August 19, 2014. The same birthday as Nick! Gerry was thrilled to have a granddaughter, as was I.

———

Gerry and I went to Scotland for two weeks in July 2015. I had been before, with my mother and sisters. Gerry's family on his father's side were also from Scotland, and he had always wanted to travel there. I was happy to go back.

We flew to Glasgow, arriving at eight in the morning. Picking up a rental car at the airport, Gerry took on the right-hand drive, and I attempted to navigate using the screen on the dashboard. We drove to nearby Paisley, where my grandmother had been born. It was July 9, my mom's birthday. At supper that night, we raised a fond toast to her and to her mother, who had braved the long journey to Canada in 1912.

The next day we headed to Vindolanda, near Hadrian's Wall. Gerry had a fascination with ancient Rome, and we walked up and down the many excavation sites, followed by lunch and a tour at the Roman Army Museum. We then drove to Hadrian's Wall, where after walking a short section and taking pictures, we realized we were famished. The nearby pub was crowded, but eventually we were back in the car and heading to that night's bed and breakfast outside Jedburgh, a little over an hour away. The light was fading as we entered our room.

We were exhausted. Gerry was peevish, complaining about supper, the car, the bathroom. I listened, nodding, and suggested we watch television in bed. We both needed a good night's rest.

The next morning, he was in even worse humour. The roosters were loud, the shower was cold. Again, I just nodded. Downstairs at the breakfast table, I poured myself a glass of orange juice and asked if he would like some.

"No, I don't want orange juice," he snapped, in a voice that suggested I had offered him pig's blood.

"Orange juice is good for you," I said lightly.

In a voice full of contempt, he snarled, "I know orange juice is good for me."

The rudeness was too much. I was done.

"Fine, Gerry. I don't know what's wrong with you. But I am not going on like this. If you don't want to be with me, fine, you take the car and keep the reservations. I can manage on my own. When we're both back in Canada, we can decide what to do next." I downed my orange juice in one gulp.

As was normal in these kinds of interactions, he immediately apologized. "Oh, I'm such an idiot, please forgive me."

But I had gone beyond mere apologies. I was deeply hurt and not that curious about why he was being such a jerk. We couldn't finish the conversation, because our hosts came in and began chatting pleasantly about our travel plans. I left it to Gerry to respond and went upstairs to pack.

It's not easy to have a fight when you're on a trip. The very nature of being a couple in unusual circumstances means you have to pull together. Plus, there are so many things to comment on. Nonetheless, for the following few days I was consumed with doubt about the future of our relationship. I loved Gerry to pieces, but I was not going to spend my remaining years with a rude, crabby man, especially one who was professionally charming to everyone else. It never once occurred to me that we always had the option of seeing a relationship counsellor when we got home, which is puzzling, since so many of my Buddhist retreats featured exercises in "having difficult conversations." Gerry worked very hard to get back on my good side, including remaining calm and non-judgmental when I sideswiped a car mirror while driving on the left.

Eventually we were back on our usual footing, enjoying the sights and scenery and amusing each other with jokes and observations. But I was wary. Was Gerry changing? Had the car accident, now seven years in the past, caused some sort of alteration in his personality? Or was it a crisis of middle age, a slow descent into a state of discontent?

Our last night in Scotland, we again stayed in Paisley. At supper that night, I wore a newly purchased paisley shawl and my mom's pearl earrings and necklace in her honour. Later, in our room, suitcases covering the bed as we packed to return to Canada, my phone buzzed—a text from sister Gail. I read it out to Gerry.

July 22, 2015, 12:07 a.m.

—Didn't want to upset you on your last few days of holidays. Last evening Dad had a seizure, and we got him to the hospital via ambulance. Dad is very lucid and seems to be coping well. The hospital staff are amazed at how well he is doing for a ninety-year-old.

"I'm sorry," Gerry said. "What do you want to do?"
"I have to go," I said. "I'll let Gail know."

July 22, 2015, 12:30 a.m.

—I'm feeling sort of teary. I will look into coming tomorrow.

After we arrived in Halifax the next day, Gerry continued on to St. John's, and I flew to Ottawa. Dad had been discharged from hospital by the time I arrived. Gail, Robin, and Jan were there. It was just over a year since we had been together, looking after our mother, and we soon fell back into the routine. As a Second World War veteran, Dad was allotted more nursing care than Mom had, and this gave us more personal time.

An email to a friend:

Saturday, August 20, 2016

This is a tremendous help to us, as it is painful to watch a parent decline, and of course there are many memories of caring for Mom in similar circumstances. So we are sad a lot. Dad is great, very lucid when awake and quite accepting of what is happening to him. That is almost saddest of all, as it is so unlike him!

Dad was harder to care for than Mom. I participated in two occasions when he ended up on the floor in the hallway, not conscious and barely breathing. The last time this happened, the night nurse luckily arrived and instructed us to get a sheet under him, and six of us grabbed the ends and toted him back to his bed, where he regained consciousness.

We started a Facebook group called McGee Family Updates, as the simplest way to keep everyone informed, including Nick, who was in Taiwan.

McGee Family Updates
August 31, 2015

Dad has been in bed all day. He has not eaten since yesterday at noon. He didn't even take his meds today. He can stand but not walk. Joan the nurse came by in the evening and put in a subcutaneous line so he can get his meds and pain control substances by injection instead of having to swallow them. She wanted to put in a catheter, but Dad refused. He can't go for long in this condition . . .

September 2, 2015

Well, it's just after midnight and Dad is still alive. There were a number of family members throughout the day. Dad had a brief period of responsiveness this afternoon, and all of his kids got a chance to let him know we were here. He even had a little J & B whisky via a swab! But mostly he has been peaceful.

Tonight, the rhythm and sound of Dad's breathing changed, and we settled in for a vigil, but he is still not ready to go. However, according to the nurse, he is in the last stage, but that can go on for some time. And so we wait. Love to all.

September 2, 2015

Robert Stronge McGee passed away at 8:30 this morning, September 2. He had a peaceful death. More details to follow.

Gerry flew up for the memorial service, which was held in the family living room and was for both of my parents. A few days later, my siblings and I scattered their ashes in the Ottawa River.

That fall I inherited a substantial sum, as did all my six siblings. A gift from my dad the accountant, who lived as if it was still the dirty thirties ("Don't throw out that half-slice of bread; we can use it for something!"). Gerry and I were astounded and grateful, full of the conflicting emotions that arise as a result of benefiting from the death of a loved one.

Gerry and I made a list of places we would like to visit and paid off some of our debts. We gave Nick and Chris a large sum, so they could share in Dad's legacy. We wanted them to have the money when they were young, because that's when expenses are plentiful, especially if you have kids. Also, that way we could squander the rest with a clear conscience.

On December 17, 2015, Nick returned from Toronto, where he was working on his doctorate. Caitlin Henry, a young woman he had been seeing for over a year, joined us a few days before Christmas. We had a lovely holiday season, introducing Caitlin to our family and babysitting the grandchildren on New Year's Eve. Before they returned to Toronto on January 3, Gerry and I took Nick and Caitlin, along with Chris and Maggie, for the tasting menu with wine pairing at The Reluctant Chef. It was wonderful—the clink of dishes, the taste of wine, exquisite flavours, and all in the company of our beloved sons and their loving partners. We had it knocked.

"Wow," said Gerry afterwards, "that's the most expensive restaurant bill I've ever paid." We smiled at each other, delighted to be able to treat our children and ourselves.

The inheritance raised some questions, though. I texted my sister.

January 27, 2016, 2:58 p.m.

—I went to the bank last week, but we didn't make any decisions. We are going back on Feb. 1 to talk with a financial advisor. I'm not sure if I want to put money into a tax-free savings account in Gerry's name. Does that sound terrible? I'm also not sure I want to pay off all our mortgages. It makes sense if we stay married forever, but what if we don't?

—My advisor says they never recommend paying off a

mortgage with an inheritance, just in case of divorce.
I didn't make any decisions yet either.

February 2, 2016, 3:42 p.m.

– We went to the bank again, and I spoke about not wanting
to put much more into matrimonial assets just in case of
marriage breakdown. Gerry and the young male advisor
were somewhat shocked! But I've already put $100,000
into household debt.

I felt unable to tell Gerry that my caution over the inheritance sprang from his behaviour in Scotland the previous summer. We were never good at discussing our relationship. Perhaps it was because of the 1988 Terms of Union, when we agreed not to talk about what happened during the time we were split up. I'm sure I referred to earlier boyfriends from time to time over the years, but only as they figured in stories I was telling—never in any emotional history kind of way. And I never asked Gerry for the details of his earlier relationships.

This is not surprising, I guess. Compared to the daily concerns of raising two children and keeping financially solvent, events that happened years ago are not important. But even though the kids were grown and gone, and even though I was curious, I did not ask Gerry any questions when he told me in September 2015 that he had received an AA apology from Mary.

———

My sister Gail was scheduled to have a knee replacement, and I was going to Ottawa to assist her. But first, I went to a Shambhala program in Patzcuaro, Mexico, from February 24 to March 6, 2016.

I had never been to Mexico before and was a little nervous. But the small town was lovely, and I felt safe to walk around during our break times. The weather was balmy, so comforting after the Canadian cold. Gerry and I texted frequently, and I deluged him with photos of exotic flowers and trees. We began to plan a fall trip to Barcelona.

And when I returned from Mexico, he was acting a little strangely.

———

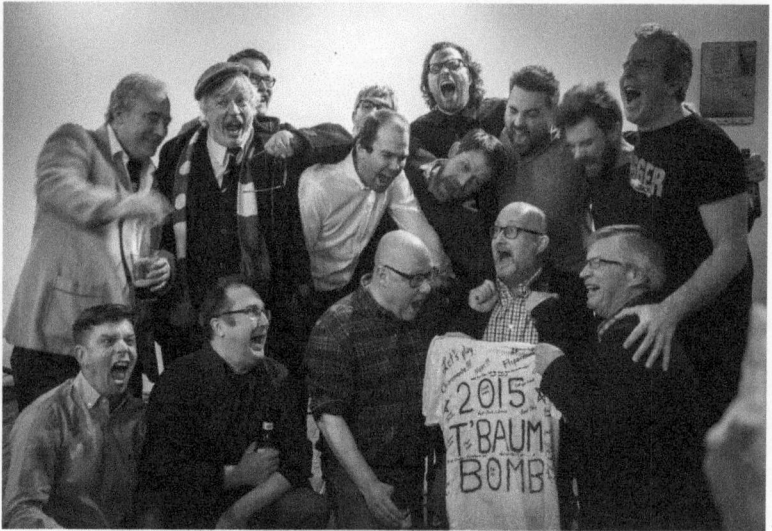

NINE

Gerrypalooza was over. It was eleven p.m. and most guests had left. The Rocket staff were cleaning up, prepping for the morning's photography class. Nick wheeled Gerry to the private bathroom and came out ten minutes later, saying he needed my help. Inside Gerry was very weak, and very upset, with urine soaking his jeans. I had seen his glass refilled several times during the night, and I immediately assumed he'd had too much to drink. Plus he was exhausted. We needed to get him home as soon as possible.

Nick was angry about the people who had been refilling Gerry's glass all evening. "How could those idiots think it was a good idea to give him all that wine?"

It took the two of us to get Gerry off the toilet and into the wheelchair. Paul had expertise in these matters and was able to transfer him from the wheelchair into the car.

"Do you want me to meet you at your house?" he asked.

"No, that's all right, there's three of us, we can manage," I replied.

Caitlin drove right to our house, and with great difficulty, Nick and I got Gerry out of the car and through the front door. He could not stand, even with his cane, and had to crawl up the stairs on his knees, swearing like a trooper as his wet jeans began to fall off. We followed closely. It was agonizing. "I hate this, I hate this," he said. "I hate you guys."

"No, you don't," I murmured, "this is just really hard."

Finally, Gerry was next to the bed, and Nick and I hoisted him up to sit on the edge. I gently pushed him onto his back and began to remove his wet clothes. Suddenly, his eyelids fluttered and his eyes rolled back.

"He's having a seizure," Nick and I said simultaneously, but as soon as we had uttered those words, Gerry was conscious again.

He had never had a seizure before. I again assumed it was due to excessive alcohol interacting with his various medications.

Somehow we got him to drink some water, took his clothes off, put his pyjamas on, and settled him to sleep. Just in case, I decided to stay awake and keep an eye on him, propping myself up in bed beside him.

Predictably, Gerry felt terrible the next day, nauseous and with a dreadful headache. Nick and I tried to get him to drink water, believing he was dehydrated from the alcohol.

"I wonder why I feel so awful."

"I know why," I said. "You had a ton to drink last night."

"I don't know if it's that," he replied dubiously.

People were deluging Facebook with their gratitude at being part of Gerrypalooza. I was kept busy on the laptop, "liking" all their remarks and reading them to Gerry as he lay under the duvet.

λ Friday night was as spiritual as any gathering I've ever attended. Honoured to have been there. Honoured to have

known the man and the mind and the wit. Time isn't holding
up. Time isn't after us. Same as it ever was. Same as it ever
was. Cheers, Gerry.

θ Tonight I was reminded of the sheer strength and love that
this community possesses. It is deep. It is never ending.
Thank you, Gerry and Debbie.

Φ Thank you so very much for all the love, loving, kindness,
clarity, joy, sadness, sharing, truth, and beauty. I am forever
transformed.

Ψ What a party it was! The crowd of friends and family, the
song, the slide show, the tributes, the tears, the laughter,
and Ursula in her yellow boots. Thank you all so much!

✳ What a wonderful night . . . Thank you to all the Porters and
McGees for an amazing evening . . . So much love . . . xox

"Those are lovely," Gerry murmured. I looked forward to sharing
our thoughts on Gerrypalooza, when he was better and I was
less exhausted. But for now I had to nap, lying down beside
him.

At 3:30 that afternoon, Chris (tenor sax) and Maggie (violin)
were playing in Duane Andrews's Earhart Ensemble at the
Factory, a large music venue on Water Street. I had invited my
sister Gail, brothers Jim and Mark, and sister-in-law Debbie to
attend. It was obvious Gerry could not go, and Nick elected to
stay home and keep an eye on him. When I returned around
five o'clock, Gerry was awake but still in bed. He had not eaten
and did not feel any better.

That night, we were having a supper party for the out-of-town relatives, most of whom were leaving the next day. So while lasagna (courtesy of two friends and M&M) and wine were being consumed by ten or so people in the living room, Nick, Chris, Lisa, and I spent most of the evening upstairs with Gerry, theorizing about what to do. Caitlin travelled back and forth between the two rooms. When I did visit downstairs, I was pleased to see my brothers in a lively debate with Gerry's dad, and my sister and sister-in-law laughing and telling stories with Gerry's cousins.

Gerry was in no shape to go downstairs and visit. He was now sick to his stomach, and around nine o'clock, Lisa went out to buy some Gravol and Alka-Seltzer, which he also threw up. Luckily, Lisa had a high school friend who was a doctor with experience in palliative care, and she arranged a phone call for me.

Wrapped in a sweater, I crouched on the cold floor in my dark back porch, back against the door. I could barely hear the happy crowd of McGees and Porters in the living room. Holding the phone to my ear, I explained to the doctor about Gerrypalooza, the seizure, and my theory about too much alcohol.

"When did he start throwing up?" she asked.

"A couple of hours ago."

"Not last night?"

"No."

"Generally, people who are sick from alcohol start throwing up immediately."

The seizure and the headache and the nausea led her to believe that his state was due more to the tumour, rather than any amount of alcohol he had consumed.

I wondered if we had shortened his life by holding Gerrypalooza. "Maybe we shouldn't have done it."

She disagreed. "Or maybe it prolonged his life. He might have been hanging on for the party, and the physical exertion of the event drained the last of his energy reserves. You will never know."

That all made sense. I asked myself why I had not taken the seizure more seriously. I thought of myself as a realist, but apparently even I could be in denial.

The doctor suggested I call the Palliative Care Unit. I thanked her profusely and walked upstairs, glad to be back in the warm.

Gerry was still sleeping. I reported the conversation with the doctor to the upstairs team of Nick, Chris, and Lisa. Nick felt we should take Gerry to emergency.

"No," I said. "Emerg will be a nightmare for him. You know what it's like there. And with the do not resuscitate order, what treatment can they offer?"

"But last night he was fine!" Nick said. "He ate Indian food and partied all evening! There has to be something they can do for him!"

"If he gets admitted, he might end up dying there. Gerry wants to die at home unless we can't manage. If this is the beginning of the end, we have to accept it. If he goes anywhere, it will be the Miller Centre."

Nick and Caitlin left for a walk in the cold night air, and when they returned, Nick seemed resigned. "I guess we'll see how tonight goes," he said.

All the guests left by eleven o'clock, for the most part unaware of the turmoil going on upstairs. I gave Gail a private explanation of what was happening, and she offered to stay the night on the couch, in case I needed help. "No, you get some good sleep," I said. "Nick and Caitlin are here."

Back upstairs, I could tell that Gerry had to pee, as several times he got out of bed and made his way with some difficulty to our small ensuite bathroom, only to turn around once he got there, as if he had forgotten why he went in. Wondering if the toilet was too low for him, I set up the commode beside the bed. But no matter how I tried to explain its use, nothing seemed to make sense to him.

"I don't know how to help you," I said. He got back in bed. It was around midnight, just twenty-four hours since Gerry-palooza ended.

Later that night things took a turn for the worse. As I dozed beside him, Gerry got up, making his way to the bathroom. I stayed in bed, thinking that maybe he would get better results without me there. It didn't work. I heard a crash and rushed in. He was sitting on the bathroom floor, back to the toilet, legs stretched out in front of him.

"Are you okay? Did you hurt yourself?"

"I'm fine. I can't get up."

I woke Nick. There was no physical room for us to get behind Gerry and lift him up.

"If you could bend your knees, and put your feet on the floor, we could pull you up by your arms," I suggested.

"Yeah. Okay. All right," Gerry said.

But he did not move.

"Can you do it?" I asked.

"Yeah. Okay. All right."

After a few repetitions, I realized he was not able to follow directions, perhaps not understanding me. Nick and I looked at each other. It was the middle of the night, the second evening with little sleep for either of us, and we were stumped.

We wrapped a feather duvet around Gerry and helped him curl up on the floor beside the heavy plant stand in front of the window, his head on a pillow inches from the toilet. I turned up the heat and turned off the overhead light. Gerry seemed to be asleep.

"We're already not managing," I said. "He deserves better than this."

It would take too long to arrange for Gerry to die at home. The Community Services palliative care office would not be open till Monday. Then a doctor would need to assess that Gerry was in the last month of his life before we could get any nursing care. He needed help now.

Standing in the bedroom, one eye on Gerry, I called the PCU at the Miller Centre. It was two a.m. Nick sat on the bed and watched me.

I explained the situation to the nurse who answered the phone. "We will have a bed tomorrow morning," she said. "Would you like it?"

"I'm not sure. I think so. Unless something changes."

"We'll call you tomorrow morning, sometime after nine o'clock. You can decide then."

Nick went back to his room. Gerry was still sleeping, or so I hoped. I lay with my head at the foot of the bed, so I could see him. All I could think about was his poor bladder.

Morning finally arrived. Nick and I were checking on Gerry, both of us pale with exhaustion, when I got the call asking if we still wanted the bed.

"Yes, please," I replied.

"Do you want an ambulance, or are you going to bring him in yourself?"

"He's on the bathroom floor," I said, "we can't get him up."

"Oh my dear, you should have called the fire department! They would have got him up."

I was mortified. How could I not know that, after eight months of learning about this stupid illness? I knew you weren't supposed to call the ambulance for falls, and I just assumed that included the fire department.

My brother Mark and sister Gail dropped by, and I explained the situation. Gail proceeded to clean up from the lasagna party. Caitlin made coffee. She had only come for Gerrypalooza and had to return to Toronto at noon to finish teaching her university course.

The ambulance attendants rang the doorbell around ten o'clock. They were two men, one older and experienced, one young and strong-backed. They were kind and reassuring as I explained the situation on our way up the stairs. I left the room so they would have space to work. I could hear them talking. "Okay, Mr. Porter, what kinda trouble are you after getting yourself into? Let's get you up off the floor." Once Gerry was on his feet, I heard them help him use the toilet, talking respectfully to him the whole time.

I had imagined they would use a stretcher to get him outside to the ambulance, but instead they guided Gerry down our narrow staircase, strong-backed EMT in front of him and older, experienced EMT behind. Gerry was bundled in his tattered, indigo-blue terrycloth bathrobe, with a grey T-shirt and red plaid pyjama pants underneath, his feet stuffed in brown checkered slippers. A little clutch of us gathered in the downstairs hallway, willing it to go well. I looked over at brother Mark. He had never been in Newfoundland before. Seeing him in our house made the situation seem even more surreal.

The older EMT kept Gerry talking as they descended. "So Mr. Porter, did you grow up in town or around the bay?"

"In town," Gerry replied without hesitation.

"Oh yes, around here?"

"No, Wadland Crescent, East End."

"Lovely."

The journey was agonizingly slow, pausing on each step as Gerry retched, the projectile vomit spattering on the steps.

"I'll clean it up," said Gail.

"There's laundry, too," I replied. "All his clothes from Gerry-palooza."

"I can do it," she said. "Don't worry. I'm glad there's something I can help with."

Finally, they had Gerry eased on to the stretcher, which was set up on the sidewalk outside our front door, the ambulance nearby. I imagined the excitement this was causing on the street. "Would you like to come with him?" asked the older EMT. I grabbed my coat and purse.

"I'll tell Chris and Lisa," Nick called after me as I left the house.

I felt a sense of deep relief as I climbed into the ambulance and sat on a narrow bench beside Gerry's stretcher. He was going to be looked after by people who knew what they were doing. He did not seem awake, but I held his hand as we drove along Circular Road, past Bannerman Park and Government House. Five minutes later we pulled up to the front door of the Miller Centre, which was almost across the road from Chris and Maggie's house. The fresh air was bracing as I watched the EMTs wheel Gerry on his stretcher up the ramp to the main door. I followed behind, trailing them through the small front lobby to the elevators. "Almost there," said the older EMT encouragingly as the elevator door opened. A minute later we were in the PCU on the third floor. The nurses were expecting us and quickly bustled Gerry away. "The family lounge is that way," they said, pointing down the hall. I thanked the EMTs profusely.

Entering the lounge, I took in the beige couches, turquoise chairs, wooden tables, and a few early Christmas decorations. I noted a stove, a fridge, and a microwave. Not cozy, but all very functional. Piling my coat on the chair beside me, I sat at a table, half-heartedly scrolling through the many Gerrypalooza comments on Facebook. Half an hour later, a nurse showed me to Gerry's room, the first one on the left as you entered the unit. I opened the door quietly, not wanting to wake him.

Gerry was standing beside his hospital bed in a blue johnny coat, attached to the rails by a catheter. He looked at me, his brow furrowed. "What's going on?" he said. I rushed to get help.

"My heavens," said the nurse, "how did he find the energy to climb out of bed?"

Chris arrived, as did Lisa and Gerry Sr. Nick had driven Caitlin to the airport and soon joined us. We gathered around Gerry's bed, watching him sleep. In my mind, he might be there for a while, and we would need to conserve our strength.

"So how are we gonna do this?" I said. "Somebody should always be here with Gerry. I don't want him to be alone. But Nick and I haven't slept for two nights, we have to get some rest."

"Well, Dad and I can stay today," said Lisa.

"I can stay overnight," said Chris.

"Okay, we'll go home now and come back to let you go for supper," I said.

At home, Gail told us that Johnny, Gerry's dear friend from cards, had stopped by our house to visit, and she had let him know that Gerry had been taken to the hospital by ambulance. Johnny told Gail that he had been keeping an eye on Gerry's glass at Gerrypalooza, to make sure he did not get too much alcohol. *I wish I had known that*, I thought to myself. I emailed him later that night:

Sunday, November 27, 2016

Hi, Johnny. I heard Gail told you the news. Tomorrow I might make a post on Facebook. I'm gonna wait till the staff doctor sees him. I'd prefer if the news stayed small (if such a thing is possible in St. John's) till then. Although Mary S., who must have heard from Ed (who I know heard from you) just told Francine, who texted me. So, it might be too late, but I'm hoping to post myself with the facts before people start talking on Facebook and Twitter. Once I do that you can start to let people know.

Thanks a lot,

xoxo

Debbie

———

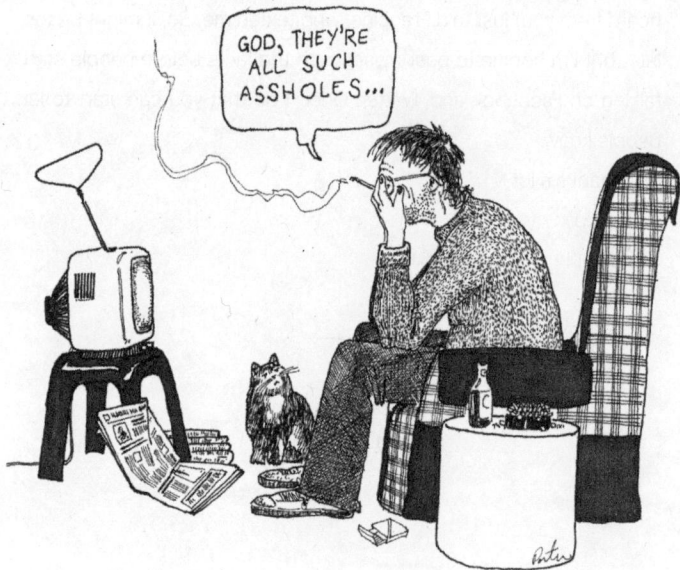

MY VERY LAST EDITORIAL CARTOON.

TEN

On November 28, 2016, I posted on Facebook:

Debbie McGee
November 28, 2016

Dear Friends,

I'm sorry to tell you that Gerry Porter has been admitted to the
Palliative Care Unit at the Miller Centre. If you want to post a
message to Gerry, please do so on the Gerrypalooza event page—
we are reading them to him when he is awake. Guess we had that
party just in time. Thanks for all the love.

One hundred and six people left comments. Here are two:

I feel very privileged to have witnessed the outpouring
of love and support for the McGee/Porter family at
Gerrypalooza. I have been to many events, but none that
were as fun/heart-wrenching/authentic as that one. You

are all magnificent and are a great example to all of us . . .
Gerry Porter, you are in our thoughts, now and always.

▶ I feel so grateful that I got to hug and talk to you on Friday
night, Gerry. You were gobsmacked with the love and in awe
of the remarkable village we get to call home. And the village
turned out in spades to honour you and say goodbye. Thank
you for giving us this invaluable memory of you and your
amazing family. Go in peace, my good man. You did well.

That day, Monday, my sister and brother left, and Gerry had his
first visit from the palliative care team of doctor, social worker,
and nurses. A cannula with an injection port was inserted into
the back of his left hand to make it easier to give medication.
There were sponges for moistening his mouth and Vaseline to
keep his lips from chapping. It was all geared to reducing any
discomfort he might feel.

Gerry's room had a view of the parking lot and the peni-
tentiary in the distance. There was a lounge chair beside the
hospital bed, and a few folding chairs for visitors. We brought
in a laptop computer and speakers, setting it up on the bedside
food table. The room was hot and dry, so I brought in a humidifier,
placing it on the windowsill. After we topped Gerry's bed with a
quilt from home and arranged a few lamps for mood lighting, the
room was much cozier.

We listened to the Gerrypalooza playlist on the laptop.
I hadn't paid much attention to the selections but now heard
that nestled amongst The Beatles, Frank Zappa, and jazz greats
were songs like "The Man Comes Around" by Johnny Cash, "Let
the Mystery Be" by Iris DeMent, and the incomparably beautiful
"The Water" by Johnny Flynn.

The water sustains me without even trying
The water can't drown me, I'm done
With my dying

By the afternoon, our closest friends had come to visit. Gerry had rallied somewhat and was able to speak with his buddies from cards and work. I did not stay in the room, wanting them to be free to express any feelings they might not want me to witness. But I accompanied them down the hall as they left, some teary, some not. The grandchildren came to visit but were not much impressed with the hospital setting and didn't stay long.

I emailed Lisa from home late that night:

Tuesday, November 29, 2016
We left at midnight when Chris arrived. He's staying the night. If Chris could leave by eight, he could help get the kids to school and daycare, so if you or your dad is available, that would be great. Nick and I will get there around ten. I'm going to stay tomorrow night, cause I have to take the car in on Wednesday and it's the only way I'll get up in time!

Gerry had a peaceful evening. We read him all the messages, and he seemed to be hearing them. Had visits from Ted, Martha, Rick, and Susan. Got an email from John P., which made him really happy.

John P. and his wife, Rosemary, were Toronto friends from Gerry's days in the student press. I had never met them. Gerry very much wanted them to know his health situation and had asked Nick to tell them about Gerrypalooza. They had not replied to Nick's email, and we couldn't find a phone number for them. I was checking Gerry's email and Facebook as I sat beside his bed and gasped with delight to find a reply from them. They had been off-grid in North Ontario.

Monday, November 28, 2016

Hello, John!

I'm so glad to get your message. This is Debbie, Gerry's wife. I'm sorry to tell you that he has just moved into palliative care. He is dozing, but when he heard me say (as I checked his email) "A reply from John P.!" he roused himself, and when I finished reading it aloud, he said, "Oh beautiful!" He had really wanted you to know what is going on with him. He can't talk for long now, so a phone call is out. But if you send a message, I will read it to him. I know you are not on Facebook, but if you call Tim, he can fill you in on recent events.

Bye for now,

Debbie

Tuesday, November 29, 2016

Hi, Debbie,

Thanks so much for replying, even though this must be an unimaginably difficult time for you. Yet I can feel Gerry's strength and warmth somehow shine through the pixels this moment. Just tell him that Rosemary and I are thinking of him, and you, during these hours and days. I'll reach out to Tim.

With all our love,

John and Rosemary

Gerry was drowsy but able to make limited conversation and did not seem in any distress. His biggest discomfort was the catheter. Based on my experience with my parents, I assumed this situation might go on for a while. We still had time.

Sister Gail, now back in Ottawa, reached out:

—Thinking about all of you. Can't stop looking at all the pics and postings from Gerrypalooza. Such love and good heartedness as only Newfoundlanders can do. I'm awed by it all. How's my *beau frère* doing today?

November 29, 2016, 9:35 p.m.

—Still hanging in. A little more stable. He hasn't eaten solid food since Friday evening. But he had some popsicle today. He doesn't talk much, but he does pay attention to what is said and sometimes responds or corrects. He loves listening to the messages. He mouths the words to songs that are playing and sometimes taps his fingers to the beat. But his chest is getting congested, and he is coughing. Trying to judge how long he has left is hard.

Gerry's first serious girlfriend, Martha, came to visit on two evenings in the middle of that week. They'd had a limited friendship in the thirty-odd years since their breakup, and I did not know her well, but she had been at Gerrypalooza and appreciated that I had referenced their relationship in my speech. I enjoyed talking with her while Gerry slumbered, telling her about our life.

Gerry's dad, who knew Martha from their shared past, came in during her second visit, and we all chatted until he suddenly broke down, crying with his head in his hands. I was on the opposite side of the bed, holding the sleeping Gerry's hand, and could not muster the energy to get up. I watched as Martha patted Gerry Sr. on the shoulder, murmuring comforting words.

That night, Wednesday, I slept on the fold-out lounge chair next to Gerry's hospital bed for the first time. We held hands through the rails. "We didn't finish season four," he said, referring to our rewatch of *Buffy* and *The Wire*. I smiled. "Oh well," I replied, "we know how they end."

When I returned the next day from taking the car to get snow tires, Gerry slept during my visit. Meals were still being delivered by the food support team, and Nick and I went home for a lamb stew and fresh bread supper. I texted Francine.

November 30, 2016, at 7:43 p.m.

—Hi, Francine,

The food delivery system is working really well. I'm not sure how long Gerry has left, but I am thinking we would like to keep up the deliveries until after the wake.

Thank you,

xo Debbie

When Nick and I returned after supper, Gerry was still sleeping, although Lisa and Chris reported that he had spoken with them before we got there. That night, as Gerry and I held hands through the bedrails, I realized that I would never get the chance to talk about Gerrypalooza with him. It was too late to discuss any of the things I had put off asking or telling him during our years together.

On Thursday, December 1, Gerry was much quieter. A poker buddy who had been out of town for Gerrypalooza came by for a visit, and Gerry did not wake up the whole time. Since Gerry had been admitted the previous Sunday, many of Lisa's friends had come to visit with her in the room, sometimes going down to the family lounge if there were two or more. Over Salvadoran chicken stew at home that night, Nick expressed discomfort that he didn't know any of her friends and was not enjoying having strangers around him at this very personal time.

"I want to feel free to cry if I want, not answer questions about my thesis topic."

"Tomorrow we'll put a sign on the door," I said, "family only."

When we returned to the hospital, a nurse took us aside in the hallway outside Gerry's room. "You should prepare yourselves," she told us. "He doesn't have long left."

Nick called Chris to tell him. He arrived shortly.

I reached out to Gail:

December 1, 2016, 7:44 p.m.

—Tonight the nurse told us within two days

That evening the boys and I sat soberly in the room. Gerry was sleeping. Astoundingly, around eight o'clock, a live brass band began loudly playing "Joy to the World." I went in search of the racket. Gathered in the social lounge right outside the PCU was the Church Lads' Brigade Regimental Band, entertaining the many patients of the Miller Centre with their annual Christmas concert. Looking past the snare drums, tubas, trombones, fifes, and bugles held by the red-coated musicians, I saw enough people sitting in rows of chairs that it did not seem possible to ask them to stop or relocate. Back in the unit, I asked a nurse how long she thought it would go on. "Probably an hour," she said. "For sure over by nine." Our evening was punctuated by drumbeats, trumpet blasts, and glockenspiel. It was absurd. I felt if Gerry was awake, he would appreciate the humour in the situation.

That night, alone at last, I abandoned the lounge chair and crawled into the hospital bed with Gerry. It had been a week since we had lain beside each other, and I relished the feel of him next to my body. I was still holding him when Nick came to replace me around nine o'clock the next morning, but Gerry did not wake up. I went home to shower, and as I was drying my hair, Nick phoned.

"The doctor says it could be any time," he said. "You should come back."

He told me that during their rounds that morning, members of the team felt that Gerry might be in discomfort, as he kept moving his legs restlessly. They made a decision to remove the catheter and to give him a small amount of morphine.

This made me sad. I did not want him to be uncomfortable, but I knew there would be little chance of talking with him again if he was on morphine. I began to regret every minute I had spent outside the hospital. "I'll be there in fifteen," I said. "Let Chris know."

"I'll tell Lisa, too," he said.

Once I arrived, there were still pragmatic things to attend to. In the family lounge, I had a tortuous conversation with someone from Memorial University's human resources department, trying to determine the cost-benefit of buying back Gerry's pension from the first year he had worked at MUN. We had investigated this before but had always put off making a decision. This would be the last chance to do so. Luckily, I was still able to perform simple math equations, and with the help of Nick's somewhat fresher perspective, decided it was not worth pursuing further.

Next, I called the funeral home—it would not be long, would they have room?

"Lots," they said.

And finally, I contacted Jan.

December 2, 2016, 2:08 p.m.

—Jan, dear, what stage is the urn at?

—Hi, Darlingest, it just needs to be varnished now. I've agonized over the finish. I could just wax it, but varnish will make it look richer, I think. Unless you are opposed to varnish? I can get it out express on Monday. Will that be okay?

—What would be faster? If you waxed it, could it be sent tomorrow? He will be cremated shortly after he dies, and we were hoping to have the urn at the visitation.

—Okay, I'll get on it 😙. You could always varnish it sometime down the road if you want. I'll get it out tomorrow for sure.

December 2, 2016, 5:52 p.m.

—Wonderful! Pick the fastest way—I will pay for speed. (Not the drug, tho)

The entire family was there at various points during the day, but by suppertime it was just me and Nick. When the evening nurse came to turn Gerry in bed and give him his meds, we walked down to the lounge, hungry for the leftover Salvadoran chicken stew we had in the fridge.

As it heated in the microwave, the nurse came down to find us.

"It will be tonight or tomorrow," she said.

Nick called Chris. He arrived quickly, around seven o'clock. The three of us sat on Gerry's bed, holding his hands, and I told them what I had learned from being present at the death of my parents. There would be changes in the colour of the skin on his feet and legs as his body shut down. There would be a long period of his breath slowing and eventually stopping. The process would take a while.

We settled in to wait, playing Gerry's music, each of us touching his hand, his arm, his chest. Absurdly, it turned out to be the night for the semi-annual power-washing of the hallway, so the sound of a large engine was omnipresent in the background. The nurses were chagrined and promised to keep them from cleaning outside our door. "Or at least out of our room," I deadpanned.

Watching Gerry sleep, we could perceive a change in the skin on his face, which somehow seemed tighter. When I checked his feet, they were turning blue. We debated whether to call Lisa. We were reluctant to add five people to our numbers. They had gone home knowing his death could be anytime. We were the core family, the four of us, and we wanted to be together for the last time. We decided not to call.

As soon as we reached that conclusion, there was a change in Gerry's breathing, as if he knew he didn't have to wait any longer.

An inhale. An exhale. A space.

"This could go on for a while," I said, and concentrated on my Buddhist practice for him, trying to hold a mind of space and clarity, joy and light.

But what do I know? Two more breaths, and he was gone.

———

I put on "Amazon Love" by Johnny Flynn, a song from Gerry's playlist he had requested for this moment.

Gonna sweep this house clean out
Gonna blow out all of the lights
We'll dream back up the Amazon
We'll steer her home tonight
We'll steer her home tonight

In the elegant sails of infinity
And the blowing winds of old love
Are the words from the mouths of the delicate crowds
In the shimmering realms up above

Blow me home, blow me home, blow me home
Take me in, hold me close, blow me home
We're aware of perspective to not be rejected
Blow me home, blow me home, blow me home

When the song was over, Nick called Lisa to tell her. "They're not coming over," he reported.

Just then a nurse came in to check on us. "He's gone," I said.

"I'm so sorry." She checked his pulse. "Take all the time you need," she said. "Take everything with you when you go."

Maggie arrived around midnight. I put on a second song, "Irish Blessing" by Ardyth and Jennifer, and as we sat silently listening, Gerry's father, Lisa, Paul, and nephews Simon and Alex entered the room, all crying. They had changed their mind. There was a period of tears and bawling and lots of hugging, and when they left, they took the sound system with them. Chris and Maggie left too, needing to relieve the babysitter, taking an assortment of blankets and pillows with them.

Nick began to pack.

I began to notify family and friends.

—He is gone. December 2 around 11:30 p.m.
Very fast and very peaceful.

The nurses said Gerry would be kept in a "room" overnight, and once a doctor had signed off on his death, he would be picked up by our chosen funeral home.

"I am going to dress him," I said. "He's not going to be cremated in a johnny coat and diaper."

I had brought his clothes with me that morning, the same ones he wore at Gerrypalooza, freshly cleaned, courtesy of my sister. As Nick schlepped load after load of green garbage bags of clothes, food, humidifiers, lamps, and laptops to our car, I struggled to dress Gerry.

Eventually Nick and a nurse came to my rescue, and Gerry looked pretty damn good on the bed when we were done. But not really like he was sleeping. There is no mistaking the difference between life and death.

It was now three in the morning, and several staff had gathered in the nursing station, all with a job to do once we vacated the room. Nick and I gave Gerry a final kiss goodbye and went home to bed in the cold night air. Unloading the car, along with everything else, would have to wait till tomorrow.

———

ELEVEN

The next evening, Saturday, December 3, Nick and I went to Chris and Maggie's for a supper of takeout fish and chips. None of us had the energy to shop or cook, but we needed to be together, maybe to declare in this small way that we were still a family, even with a core member gone.

As we sat in the living room watching the fire, Ursula, now two years and a few months, walked over to where I sat on the couch.

"Grandpa sleeping?" she asked.

Before I could formulate a careful reply, five-year-old Jack spoke up. "He's dead," he said firmly.

Ursula twisted her foot in the carpet, and said, "Maybe sleeping at hospital?"

"He's dead," Jack repeated in an even louder voice.

Undeterred, Ursula continued, "Maybe sleeping at Grandma's?"

Jack drew in a deep breath. All of us intervened at once. We were not ready to hear him shout, "He's dead!"

———

It had been a hard first day.

Waking up that morning, I had felt hollow, almost lacking in substance, as if not just a strong wind, but a strong anything, like a hearty voice, could knock me over. At the same time, I also felt a kind of resolve. The worst had already happened, so how hard could anything else be? I would not let Gerry down. I summoned the energy to keep functioning.

The wake had to be arranged, the obituary sent out, and there were messages to respond to. Gerry had only died the night before, but there were already at least fifty posts on Facebook. I considered it my duty to read and "like" each one of them.

Nick posted on Facebook. It included something I did not know.

✸ Nicholas McGee
December 3, 2016

Dad decided not to give a speech at his party, but he told me on several occasions that if he did, all he could think to say would have been a paraphrase of Lou Gehrig's famous 1939 speech to a packed audience at Yankee Stadium, after being diagnosed with his terminal illness. "People think I've been given a raw deal," Dad would say, imitating the sound of the microphone echoing across the field, "but I consider myself the luckiest man on the face of the earth."

The funeral home director called me. Gerry and I had pre-purchased three visitation sessions for the wake. When would I like to begin?

Today was Saturday. Tomorrow was Jack's fifth birthday party. I decided starting on Monday evening would give us enough time to get ready.

"We expect to be able to do the cremation later on today," he said. "Would you like to be present?"

I did not want Gerry to be alone during the cremation. What if his consciousness was hovering around somewhere? It could be frightening, or at the very least puzzling, to see himself put into an oven. I figured if he saw me there as well, it would be reassuring.

"I'll call you when we're ready," the director said. "Probably around four o'clock. And also, if you send the obituary soon, we can get it in tomorrow's paper."

I had drafted the obituary with input from Gerry as part of The Sad List. Now all I had to do was add in the date of death and put in the dates and times for the visitations.

It is with great sadness we announce the passing of Gerry Porter on December 02, 2016, after a bewilderingly short journey with brain cancer. Predeceased by his mother, Ida Healey Porter, and his mother- and father-in-law, Janette and Robert McGee. Leaving to mourn his wife, Debbie McGee, and sons Nicholas (Caitlin) and Christopher (Maggie), and his beloved grandchildren, Jack and Ursula; father Gerry Porter Sr. (Jill), sister Lisa (Paul), and nephews Simon and Alex; and half-brothers Jonathan, David, and James; and a large assortment of Healey and Porter cousins and McGee in-laws. Gerry will be missed by his colleagues at MUN's Centre for Innovation in Teaching and Learning, his buddies from cards, and his life-long friend Ed Riche. We thank the many friends who were there for us in the past eight months—and the many family members who came to visit during the period that Gerry called "The Long Goodbye." Our gratitude to Drs. Stuckless and Laing at the Bliss Murphy Cancer Centre, and Dr. Bill Eaton, Rhonda Brophy, and the many wonderful staff members of the palliative care /

pain and symptom management team at the Miller Centre. We also wish to thank the many kind but unheralded employees of Eastern Health, all of whom made this difficult time easier to bear. Cremation has taken place, and a visitation will be held at Carnell's Funeral Home, 329 Freshwater Road, on Monday, December 5 (7–9 p.m.) and Tuesday, December 6 (2–4 and 7–9 p.m.). Flowers gratefully accepted. An award celebrating Gerry's love of music will be established. Those who wish to donate at this time can make out a cheque to The Gerry Porter Award for Creative Improvised Music and mail it to 13 William Street, St. John's, NL, A1C 2S2. In accordance with Gerry's wishes, there will be no funeral service, but we thank all those who attended Gerrypalooza, Gerry's final party. Hup! Hup!

Minutes after sending this, I rushed off to Carnell's. The funeral director showed me into the cremation room, which was large and sparsely furnished, as it was not a public space for visitors. Across the empty floor, a coffin-shaped plywood crate sat on a lift, next to a curtained wall. I felt relieved to be in the same room as Gerry again.

"Would you like to see him?" asked the funeral director. I hadn't realized this was an option. I watched as he removed a large wood screw from each of the corners of the coffin and lifted off the lid.

Inside was Gerry, looking very dapper but a little cramped for space, and encased in what looked like a giant shower cap—the kind of thing we would have laughed at together. *You should see this, Gerry,* I thought to myself. *Or maybe you can.*

I was left alone with him, and during that time I told Gerry what was going on. "So, you died, Gerry, and you're going to be cremated in a short while. I'll keep you company."

The funeral home director returned ten minutes later. I watched as he resealed the coffin and then pulled back the curtains to reveal a large oven door and an impressive control panel. *Kind of like the Wizard of Oz*, I thought to Gerry, stifling an urge to giggle. The lift was raised to reach the door of the crematorium, and the coffin, with Gerry in it, slid inside.

Apparently, it can take up to five hours to cremate an adult. I sat alone in the stark room for an hour or so. I was not sad or crying; instead it felt right. I was where I wanted to be, with Gerry. I didn't want to overdo the Buddhism funeral rituals, out of respect for Gerry's atheism, but I said the *Heart Sutra* and repeated the Sukhatavi chant of *Namo Amitabhaya Hri* while occasionally reminding Gerry that he was dead and was being cremated. Just in case.

When I was ready to leave, I found the funeral director. "My sister has carved an urn for Gerry, but it just got sent today. It might not arrive in time for Monday night."

He assured me that was not a problem. "You can use one of ours until it gets here."

It was time to head to Chris and Maggie's. I picked up Nick on the way. "How was it?" he asked me. "You okay?"

"It was good," I replied. "I'm really glad I was there."

When we got home around nine o'clock, I went to my computer, intending to post the obituary on Facebook before going to bed. I was shocked to discover it had already been shared! Shouldn't that be left to me? How did someone get hold of it?

An online search showed me that the funeral home had posted the obituary on their website earlier that evening. I had forgotten that was part of their service. Someone had found it and shared it on their Facebook page.

I felt so invaded, so threatened, that even though I was exhausted, I immediately changed my Facebook profile picture (which had been a 2008 photo of me and my mother and sisters in Scotland) to two pictures of Gerry and me sitting together. One was from January 1987. The other had been taken in October 2016. I felt the need to demonstrate to the world that we had been sitting beside each other for decades.

The next afternoon, Sunday, December 4, I posted the obituary on Facebook myself, along with the following:

Debbie McGee

December 4, 2015

I wrote the majority of this obit about a month ago, based on discussions with Gerry. Yesterday there were just a few details to add. I emailed it to Carnell's for publication in Monday's *Telegram*. I was going to post it to Facebook but wanted to get to Carnell's to be with Gerry during cremation. When I returned, I was shocked to see the obituary had already been posted and shared a continually escalating number of times. Not sure why I felt that—part of the loss, maybe. He was Dad, and he was ours. Now he belongs to everyone. I guess he always did.

The post immediately received many consoling comments. I was mollified when the woman who had posted the obituary, and who privately apologized to me via email, posted:

Oh Debbie, Gerry truly was yours and we were just lucky that you shared him with us all these years, especially in recent months! Your family has been so generous during such a difficult time, and it is easy for us to forget that the loss is unique to you, Nick, Chris, and family.

At six o'clock that evening, Jack had his fifth birthday party at a children's gym. It was the first time since we had been at Gerry's bedside that the entire family had gathered. Gerry's dad was taking pictures, the rest of us eating cake and chatting with parents as happy children tumbled about on mats. I found for the first of many times that it is possible to laugh and appreciate life, even while holding an immense grief.

I was now beginning to understand where my possessive feelings had come from. On the Gerrypalooza Facebook page, many of Gerry's friends from his student newspaper days at *The Muse* had veered off-topic. While initially the photos and anecdotes had been related to Gerry, it had gradually devolved into a *Muse* reunion. That was bearable, but after he died, there seemed to be a kind of competition as to who knew and loved him best, with little consideration shown to his family. For a while, I gamely tried to participate, but then I gave up. They were having a kind of party online. My partner of thirty years was dead. I kept "liking" remarks, but I no longer meant it.

That night I texted my friend Susan McConnell on Canada's West Coast:

December 5, 2016, 2:28 a.m.

—It's funny, but I'm starting to get annoyed by all these old friends of Gerry's from thirty-five years ago telling stories about him on Facebook. It feels like a contest. Trying to analyze why I'm feeling jealous and a bit possessive. Maybe because they don't mention me or the kids. I feel like saying, yeah, if he was such a big part of your life, how come I never saw you in the past thirty years? Some old girlfriends have posted so many times about Gerry on

Facebook that I'm starting to feel weird about it. I want him
to ourselves again, although I know that's never going to
happen. Is this part of grieving?
—I'm happy with a certain amount of claiming loss,
but when anyone has posted more than a few times,
I feel personally threatened. No, it was me that he loved!
He was mine! Hard to admit I have these possessive
feelings, but I do.

Her perspective was interesting:

—Sometimes I feel like people want to get in on it,
somehow. And they are probably people who cared for
Gerry and want to feel less loss by pointing out their
importance. Doesn't work, and is hurtful to you, but
I think that's the attempt.

There was one post on Facebook that I felt did a good job in artic-
ulating the emotional impetus behind the less tactful posts. And
I found it comforting:

✦ The day before yesterday, I lost a friend, an important
friend. His name is Gerry Porter, and I met him when
I was at Memorial University working on the student
newspaper, *The Muse* . . . First and foremost, I am deeply
mourning Gerry's loss . . . But I'm also grieving everything
I left behind when I left St. John's so many years ago,
companions and fellow travellers, with whom I shared such
deep personal bonds. They are irreplaceable. I will miss
Gerry, for sure, and I also miss my friends.

I have more to say about social media, death, and grieving in the afterword.

———

Getting ready for the wake on Monday night involved minimal work but still kept us busy. I reorganized the video presentation from Gerrypalooza, creating two shows—one of personal photos and one of Gerry's artwork—and transferred each of them to compact discs. We had been assigned the downstairs section at the funeral home, including a foyer and two rooms, one larger than the other. We decided the personal photos would be shown in the main room, using the funeral home's wall-mounted screen, but a second computer and monitor had to be procured from Paul and brought into the smaller room. We printed cards for those who might want to donate to the music award and set them up in the foyer, next to the guest book. Floral arrangements kept arriving, and we were touched by the number, and by the variety. The smell of roses, freesia, and lilies filled the room.

The urn from my sister Jan was still in transit, and we chose a horizontal mahogany box as a temporary substitute. This was set up on a table at the front of the main room, where a coffin would usually go. What to display beside the urn? We settled on Gerry's grey plaid cap, which he had worn both indoors and out since 2012; one of his black recipe binders to signify his love of cooking and nurturing others; and, of course, his iPhone, all surrounded by flowers.

Amid these preparations on Monday, Lisa called to say Ed Riche was going to be interviewed about Gerry on the local CBC afternoon show at four o'clock. I remember thinking, *Are they allowed to do that without asking me?* Coming so soon after my fruitless attempt to assert control on Facebook, it was an unwelcome reminder that what I had actually lost was not control, but Gerry.

I texted with Gail:

—Caitlin is coming—she and Nick and I will go to Heart's Content maybe Thursday or Friday. I'm liking having the opportunity to cry. Nick and I are alternating between cheerful chatting and bawling.

The wake that first night was from seven to nine. It was a strangely party-like affair where I was possessed with a wild energy, like being manic but while underwater. The rooms were crowded with people, and many of them wanted to speak with me. I received many hugs, which acted as a kind of fuel source and kept me going. Guests stood and watched the video presentation of Gerry's artwork. It was like watching the past twenty years of arts-community history in the form of posters. Most were from plays, but there were also films, book covers, circus shows, musical events, dance festivals, and television series. Even I was awed, and I had lived with Gerry when he created most of them. There were close to a hundred. Where did the time go?

Nick and I returned home from the wake around ten o'clock, exhausted. I foolishly checked Facebook. There was a post on Gerrypalooza, asking if there were plans to collect and donate Gerry's graphic work to the Centre for Newfoundland Studies. I was incensed. The Facebook collective was not in charge of his legacy! It seemed to me more evidence that his university friends were completely unaware that Gerry had lived an entire life since they had known him, one that included a wife and two grown children. I replied tersely, "We're on it."

The urn from my sister arrived in time for the second and final day of the wake on Tuesday, which included an afternoon and an evening session. Gerry's ashes were transferred to the beautifully carved aspen container. It was rectangular, nine inches tall and seven inches wide, and all four sides and the base were covered with intricate, burned-in Celtic knots, with repeating motifs of interlaced lines and geometric shapes. On the wooden top, burned in using Charles Rennie Mackintosh font, was *Gerald Cameron Porter, 1962–2016*. Gerry would have loved it. It looked beautiful on the table, where Wallace Ryan, a cartooning friend from Gerry's adolescence, had brought in a drawing pencil to join the grey cap, recipe binder, and phone.

Sweetly, as is done for every MUN employee who dies:

Memorial University's flags will fly at half-mast on Tuesday, Dec. 6, from 1 to 4 p.m. to mark the passing of Gerald Porter, an employee of the Centre for Innovation in Teaching and Learning.

Since that was the same time as our wake, we didn't visit the flags at half-mast, but brother-in-law Paul took a photo and posted it on Facebook.

The last two sessions of the wake were the same energetic affairs as the night before. At the last session, Gerry's father sat on the couch in the main room, conversing with Ed's dad, his neighbour from fifty years ago. I reflected on how much change they had seen over those years, and how much loss: wives, siblings, and now for Gerry Sr., a son.

At the end of the last session, almost everyone but family gone, two musician friends came in, fresh from a performance.

As they examined the pages of the recipe binder, they confided in me that they too were about to lose a loved one. It helps to know you're not alone.

I was relieved to have the public mourning finished and was looking forward to retreating to sanctuary in Heart's Content. But first, we had to load up the cards, the guest book, the food, the photographs, the computer and monitors, endless flower arrangements (which we divided among us), and of course, the urn. Now that it held Gerry's ashes, it seemed to have achieved a certain sentience. I held it on my lap as Nick piloted the car home. All the houses and businesses were decorated for Christmas. When did that happen?

The amount of media attention that Gerry's death received surprised me. On December 6, on the front page of the *Telegram*, there was a small colour headshot of Gerry on the front page, under which was written *Gerrypalooza prize*, encouraging readers to go to the main story on page A6. There, next to the popular obituary section (where Gerry's obit was still running), was an interview with Chris on The Gerry Porter Award for Creative Improvised Music.

The article features a four-by-four, black-and-white photo of Gerry, with a bold black headline underneath: *Family creates music award in memory of Gerry Porter*. Journalist Tara Bradbury describes Gerry as "a local writer and artist, among other things, who was known on social media for his wit and his commentaries." Chris is quoted: "He was always looking for the weird and the wonderful. He really enjoyed the Sound Symposium and Night Music at The Ship. The idea behind the award is to celebrate that." Our home address is given for anyone wishing to contribute. Chris explains that so far, donations have come from "people who knew [Gerry] in real life and online." Chris is further quoted as saying, "People have been saying they will miss his generosity and his humour. Some people have said the Internet will be a lot more boring from now on."

As well, that week our local MHA, Lorraine Michael, read a statement in the House of Assembly, which was also shared on Facebook and YouTube.

I rise today to honour a remarkable person taken from us much too soon. Gerry Porter died last Friday just eight months after his brain cancer diagnosis.

The many facets of his life are reflected on Gerrypalooza, a Facebook page that began as an invitation to an event and became a page of memories and love when he moved to palliative care and now stands as a beautiful tribute.

He edited The Muse, worked as a graphic artist at Memorial, introduced people to new music and ideas, designed posters for dozens of local shows, and impressed everyone he met with his wit, wisdom, and intelligence. He was best known, lately, for his brilliant political shareables. Many of us in this House have been his subjects on social media, Mr. Speaker. But I am sure we can all agree that Gerry always avoided low blows and made us laugh at ourselves.

Most important, he was a loving husband, father, grandfather, and friend. We all feel his loss, but I send an extra big hug to Debbie, Nick, Chris, and all the other Porters and McGees.

I ask all honourable Members to join me in saluting Gerry Porter, an unmatchable example of a life well lived.

Thank you, Mr. Speaker.

The media coverage even went national. On December 12, Tom Power, host of *Q* on CBC Radio (did you know he's from

Newfoundland?), opened his show by saying, "A great artist from Newfoundland has passed," before going on to reference Gerrypalooza and ending with the importance of telling our dear ones that we love them, before it's too late.

And then, two days before Christmas, a third of a page in the *Globe and Mail*, written by Joan Sullivan. The subhead was *Gerry Porter, Newfoundland Arts Figure, 54*, and the headline was *Popular artist held a premortem party*. A colour photo of Gerry was nestled among five column inches, along with this lovely paragraph: "Sharp-witted and sweet-tempered, Mr. Porter tended to keep the friends he made: his weekly poker game went back three decades."

The article began this way:

> Newfoundland graphic artist Gerry Porter, who died this month, was known for his endless versatility. He became a prominent member of the St. John's arts community, drawing comics and designing posters and other promotional material for theatre, dance, and film productions. He also contributed to many local art projects.
>
> Mr. Porter was 54 when he died on Dec. 2, eight months after he was diagnosed with brain cancer. His death came exactly one week after a "premortem" party, dubbed Gerrypalooza, took place in downtown St. John's. Mr. Porter's wife, Debbie McGee, and two sons all spoke at the event, as his grandchildren raced around.

All this media coverage was overwhelming and felt a little absurd. Gerry was not famous or in any way a celebrity. I was torn between the pleasure of seeing Gerry and his contributions to the community recognized and the feeling of vulnerability engendered by having this most private and painful life event discussed in the public sphere. But I also noted that unlike most posts on Facebook, all the legacy media articles acknowledged his family, and I appreciated that recognition of our loss.

Two days after the wake ended, Nick, Caitlin, and I went to Heart's Content. We brought Gerry in his urn, settling him on the living room coffee table. I then abandoned all pretext of coping and went up to my room, where I cried endlessly on the bed.

———

I was not prepared for this moment. In the whole eight months, I had not contemplated my life after Gerry. I knew some of the cards guys had promised him they would look in on me, but Gerry and I had never discussed my future without him. Now I was floundering, the adrenalin that had been surging through me in the past eight months still there but no longer needed. I began to write.

I became obsessed with the details of Gerry's life in the time before I met him. Starting that night in Heart's Content, I texted, emailed, and visited his friends, trying to shake loose any memories they might have. I read through Gerry's Evernote diary on his computer. I dug out the boxes under our bed, combed back issues of *The Muse*, and went through the financial records of *Arts in formation* that I found in our basement. From all this, I put together a timeline of his childhood and teenage years, figuring out his first jobs and apartments and flings. I knew Gerry's life so much better now. All the things I had not asked over the thirty years, because they hadn't mattered that much, now mattered terribly. When had he been happy? When had he been sad? How badly had he been hurt when we split up before Nick's birth? Did he love me? Why was I doubting that?

Time became confusing. If Gerry's not here, is this before we met? All these women posting from his past, is he with them instead of me? Is that why he's not here? No, he's dead, you saw him in his coffin. But somehow, I kept feeling that maybe we just hadn't got to the part where we get together. I noticed that every time I prepared to leave the house, there would be a little feeling of anticipation inside. He wasn't in here, maybe he was out there? I might bump into him! As if somehow, time might swing round and we would suddenly be in sync again.

———

In February 2017, two months to the day Gerry died, I went on walkabout. I cried my way through a week in Nova Scotia, then on to Ottawa, Toronto, Cuba, Seattle, Victoria, and Vancouver. All the way I was supported by old friends and family, most of whom had known me before Gerry came into my life. It was good to be reminded that I was still a person, even without him.

I also met with several of Gerry's friends from his CUP days, relishing any details they shared about him and eagerly showing them photos of his children and grandchildren.

During the trip, I remained preoccupied with the various issues Gerry and I had not discussed, especially the events in Scotland that had left me wondering if we would continue to live together. Why did I attach such a dire storyline to a bad-tempered squabble? Why did I have so much difficulty in bringing it up for discussion? If Gerry and I had been able to discuss his crabbiness in Scotland at the time, it would have saved me a lot of stress, before and especially after he died.

There is something about interpersonal communication with our loved ones that makes it hard to get the right balance between being open and vulnerable while also protecting our tender hearts. It often feels safer to not even try. I blamed myself for my lack of trust.

Today I wonder why I put the onus of communication on myself. Why couldn't Gerry just say what was bothering him? What made initiating a bad-tempered squabble seem like a reasonable option? Perhaps he needed to see my visceral reaction to reassure himself that he could still affect me, maybe his way of knowing that I still loved him. It was probably maddening to see me respond placidly when he was trying to get a table-overturning reaction.

On April 3, 2017, I returned to St. John's, where grief and administrative chaos awaited me. The grief I managed with the wonderful counsellor from the Palliative Care Unit and also with my network of friends and family. After a particularly bad day, I told my friend Susan Shiner that I would never kill myself, because it would be too hard on my family.

"Yes," she warned, "you feel that now. But if things get worse, you could come to think of it as doing them a favour. Promise you'll call me if you catch yourself thinking that way."

Two women who had lost their husbands years earlier reached out to talk with me. I took each of them up on their offer and discovered the relief in crying with someone who doesn't need to be shielded from your grief.

The administrative chaos I dealt with by hiring a part-time assistant. She helped me make calls, cancel policies, get certificates, hire contractors for home maintenance. She got a job in her field a few weeks later, but by then I was able to manage on my own.

Donations had poured in for The Gerry Porter Award for Creative Improvised Music, and it was now fully funded. The first one would be given out in 2018.

Soon my house in town and the one in Heart's Content were being painted, foundations strengthened, floors replaced. I was using up my inheritance at a furious pace. But it kept me going. All that mattered was that something was happening.

———

Two large plaque-mounted posters of Gerry's rested against my hallway wall for the next year. One was for a children's play, *The Ogre's Purse*, and the other for *Habib's Unforgettable All-Night House Party*. They had been hung at Gerrypalooza, and I hadn't yet found the energy to take them to Heart's Content. Ursula was fascinated by them and would draw me into the hallway to discuss them every time she visited. I crouched beside her on the wooden floor as we examined them. Although she was now three, they were taller than she was.

Our conversation was always the same, with her telling me that Grandpa had made them, how there was a pirate ship on the purple poster, and that people were dancing in a house on the blue one.

In the fall of 2017, she surprised me. After her usual closing comment on the dancing, she paused, then looked at me, and said, "Grandpa is dead?"

I nodded. "Yes, honey, he is."

She looked down at the bracelet on her wrist, twirling it. Then she looked up at me. "That makes me sad."

"Me too, honey, oh, me too."

———

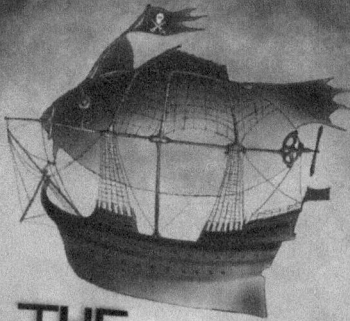

HABIB'S UNFORGETTABLE ALL-NIGHT HOUSE PARTY

LSPU HALL
3 VICTORIA STREET

JOSEPH'S STOR

JOSEPH'S LOUNGE

FEBRUARY 3-14
MATINEES:
TICKETS CALL THE HALL 752

WRITTEN BY JANET MICHAEL

RCA THEATRE COMPANY
TOURING SCHOOLS NOVEMBER 18 - DECEMBER 6, 2013

THE OGRE'S PURSE
BY PHILIP GOODRIDGE
DIRECTED BY NICOLE ROUSSEAU
FEATURING CHRIS DRIEDZIC, COLIN FURLONG, WILLOW KEAN AND CLAIRE ROULEAU

www.rca.nf.ca

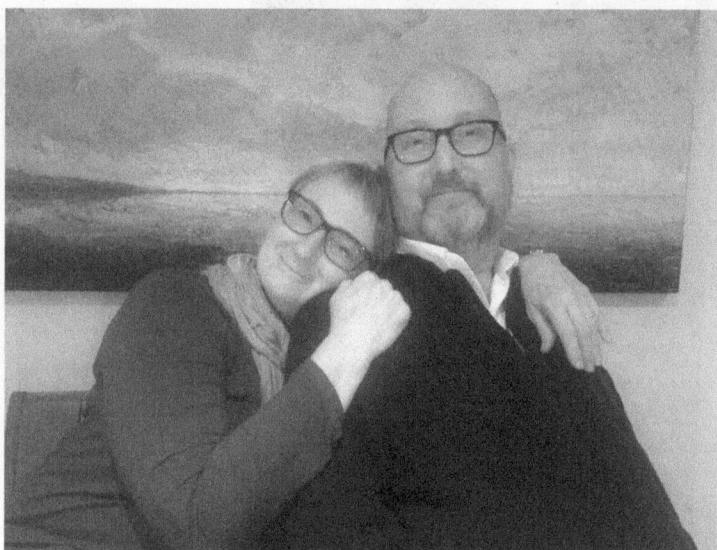

AFTERWORD

In the years since Gerry's death, I've had time to investigate my reaction to the postings on Facebook. Even a cursory search on Google will pull up many articles on death and social media.

One of the first I found was written on July 20, 2016, by Taya Dunn Johnson on Upworthy, subtitled "Grieving in the technology age is uncharted territory." The author points out that there is a hierarchy of grief, and where you stand in the hierarchy depends on your proximity to the deceased.

When someone dies, condolences are traditionally expressed in many ways. Tears, hugs, kisses, visiting, phone calls or voice messages, gifts of food or flowers, cards posted or dropped in the mailbox, attending the wake, attending the funeral. People in the inner circle might do all or most of these. It's not hard to know what is appropriate to your relationship with both the one who is gone and the ones who remain behind

But now, in the age of social media, we have additional ways of expressing grief, in the form of Facebook, X, Bluesky, and Instagram, and the hierarchy here is much less intuitive. And there are no traditions to follow.

As my grief counsellor pointed out, a post supposes an equality—anyone can participate in the virtual world. But the death has taken place in the real world, where there is no equality. No matter how seminal the deceased was in their past, the loss felt by pals from long-gone days is not equal to the loss experienced by current close family and friends.

They are mourning a loss of youth, the loss of innocence and good times. We are mourning a husband and a father, who died in our arms a few days ago. If they were in a room with us, this difference would be very clear to them.

The dying are stars to some, and many want to be associated with celebrity. Constant posting confers a legitimacy on grief that may not actually correspond to real life. A colleague with a large number of followers on Facebook posted so often that they received hundreds of condolences on Gerry's death. We were not mentioned once. To imagine my feelings, picture a similar situation happening in person. The grieving family standing by the coffin, while a lineup of strangers snakes out the door, giving condolences to a workmate of your loved one.

I understand, we're all navigating the new, reinventing the grief wheel on social media. But some things haven't changed. The family still needs to be respected. The loss of a loved one removes your skin, leaves you tender and vulnerable, and even well-meaning people can cause unintended pain.

For example, Nick was horrified and angry when his very personal and heartfelt tribute to his dad on Facebook was found by someone he didn't know and who therefore didn't have the right to share his post. Instead, they copied and pasted it on their page, and it was now able to be shared by their friends, all of whom were strangers to Nick. Because his name was on the post, every one of the reactions came to his attention.

"What the? Who *is* this person?"

"Oh, a friend of Dad's from *The Muse*. They live in BC, I think."

Our experience is echoed in an article Claire Wilmot wrote in *The Atlantic*, following the death of her sister Laura. She recounts that Laura's close friends and extended relatives learned of her death from a Facebook post by a high school acquaintance who hadn't seen Laura in years, but happened to work in the hospital where Laura died. The immediate family hadn't yet had time to make phone calls. Wilmot wrote:

At my most cynical, I wondered if posts about other people's deaths are used no differently than other content on social media—as a means of identity assertion in a busy online environment. ("The Space Between the Mourning," The Atlantic, *June 8, 2016*)

In an online *Reader's Digest* article by Alison Caporimo, Levi Williams recounts what happened when his wife died suddenly, two weeks after giving birth to their first child, Lily.

As Lily and I waited at the hospital for my family to pick us up, I was looking at my phone and noticed friends were already commenting about Lori's death on her Facebook page: "I can't believe it" and "I miss you already" were the most common. It was really disturbing. I wanted to delete the page then and there, but I had forgotten her password.

When we got home, the first thing I did was to get on her computer—which was still logged in to her Facebook account—and delete the page. It just felt like the right thing to do. She was really into Facebook and other social media. It was so her. I felt like if she wasn't there, it shouldn't be there either.

I also felt so helpless about Lori's death. I didn't want to stand by while other people took over her page with their comments and pictures—I wanted to have some control. ("Coping with Death on Facebook," Reader's Digest)

There is much we don't know about our friends and acquaintances. People live complicated lives, full of regrets, anxieties, and unresolved situations. When someone dies, all that long history is at play along with current daily life events, and they come together, sometimes in a coherent and sometimes in a clashing manner.

I've shared our personal situation to help illustrate how these complications float close to the surface after the loss of a loved one. A thoughtless comment can make it harder for the survivors to keep from going under. As we all find our way to an etiquette for death and grieving on social media, we need to be sensitive.

As Taya Dunn Johnson suggests in her Upworthy article:

If we each adopted a little patience and restraint in this area, we would help those who are in the darkest hours of their lives by not adding an unnecessary layer of stress.

Please pause and consider your role and relationship to the newly deceased. Remember, hierarchy refers to your status and your relative importance to the deceased.

If the person is married, let the spouse post first.

If the person is "young" and single, let the partner, parents, or siblings post first.

If the person is "old" and single, let the children post first.

If you can't identify the family / inner circle of the person, you probably shouldn't be posting at all.

("Please read this before you post another RIP on social media," Upworthy, July 20, 2016)

Claire Wilmot echoes this:

My proposal is simple: Wait. If the deceased is not a close family member, do not take it upon yourself to announce their death online. Consider where you fall in the geography of a loss, and tailor your behavior in response to the lead of those at the center. ("The Space Between the Mourning," The Atlantic, June 8, 2016)

Social media is now part of how we communicate with each other. And death isn't going anywhere, either. In the cultural chaos, we have to learn how to integrate the two respectfully.

No matter who you are, or what you write and in what medium, be sure to include your condolences to the family, even when you're replying to a colleague, friend, or acquaintance of the deceased. Because the Facebook algorithm ensures that it *will* end up on the family's feed. "Sorry for the loss of your friend. Condolences to their family and loved ones."

And, of course, some posters did this—by my count, approximately 30 per cent. The sense of the community holding us, caring about us, was still very strong. Also, the online mourning was helpful to others, who were part of the community but living far away. Such as this post:

> ✡ I have felt blessed to be able to share part of this journey with Gerry, you, and your family with this social media connection. Peace to you all!

And I learned some things from the posters. For example, I previously had no idea of the source of Gerry's Twitter handle, @ficklesonance. A mutual friend, Kris Klaasen, wrote:

> ◇ I'm posting "A Fickle Sonance," a song by alto saxophonist Jackie McLean, in honour of Gerry Porter, a student newspaper colleague who died Friday in St. John's, NL, after a short bout of brain cancer. I shared office space with Gerry and his CUP colleagues in 1983–84 in Ottawa. We reacquainted on Facebook where he displayed his wicked wit, insight, and kindness. Heartfelt condolences to his partner, Debbie McGee, their two sons and two grandkids. Just a short, fifty-four-year stint on the planet. The world could have used a lot more Gerry.

Many messages were from people who only knew Gerry from his online life on either Twitter or Facebook. This one was from a follower who reposted Gerry's very popular "All the Single Mussels in the Corner," which is Beyoncé's music video for "Single Ladies (Put a Ring on It)" set to an all-accordion version of a Newfoundland folksong. It is inexplicably hilarious.

> ▼ For (and by) Gerry Porter, whom I only knew peripherally but who influenced my idea of what it means to be a contemporary Newfoundlander and Labradorian.
> His wit was sharp and his heart was big. Not a bad thing to understand about a person you didn't really know.
> Rest and frolic in peace, Gerry.

I received a traditional sympathy card in the mail from an older friend of ours who was now living in Australia. She wrote, *"Since I first learned of Gerry's illness months ago, you have been in my thoughts, and I have been grateful for all the photos and messages posted on Facebook and elsewhere.*" I think of her and imagine how delighted she must have been by Gerry's jokes, his photos, and especially the posts from the community following Gerrypalooza.

Years later, I feel more compassion and understanding for what I have come to regard as social media blunders. If you choose to have such an intensely personal time in your life shared on social media, as we so clearly did, then you have to take the bad with the good.

Gerry's sense of humour and quick mind were made for social media, and I am happy he got so much pleasure out of it, especially in the last months of his life.

I believe it is a positive development that social media has increased our awareness and acknowledgement of grief and loss as part of life. The love and support, good wishes and memories that were delivered to us through Facebook during those eight months outweigh any discomfort I felt following Gerry's death. And hey, they led to this book. :)

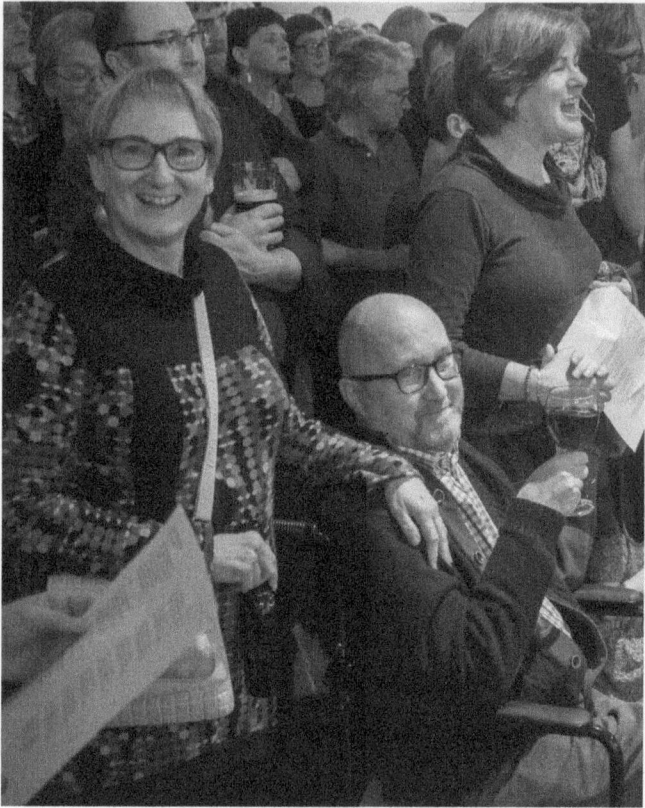

ACKNOWLEDGEMENTS

First off, I want to thank my sons for their love, courage, and support: Nick, who is now married to Caitlin, and Chris, who is now divorced from Maggie. We are all still close, because of Jack and Ursula, and there are three new people now added to the mix: Michael Collins, and my step-grandchildren Edie and Ada Collins.

Also my gratitude to my close and extended family, especially my siblings Gail, Jim, David, Mark, Robin, and Janine. And of course, Lisa Porter, the late Paul Pope, and my nephews Simon and Alex.

My friends Francine Fleming, Camille Fouillard, Jane Robinson, Genia Sussex, and Elaine Wychreschuk have always had my back, both before and after I began this project. I also want to thank Isabella St. John and the late Susan Shiner, and the arts community of Newfoundland and Labrador, particularly my own little corner of it in downtown St. John's.

My dear friend Brenda Longfellow and her wonderful partner, Glen Richards, have been with me through all the events described in this book.

In terms of writing support, I want to start with Rhonda Brophy, social worker for the Palliative Care Unit at the Miller Centre. Our discussions got me interested in writing about etiquette for online postings of death and condolences.

I attended Writing With Care, a writing retreat at Ochre Pit Cove in Newfoundland, for two years in a row, with facilitators Lois Brown, Lori Clarke, and Lisa Porter.

The incredible Lisa Moore encouraged me to continue by giving me a place in her creative non-fiction class at Memorial University. By the time the course finished, it was the first anniversary of Gerry's death.

The writing classes at MUN continued, now under the guidance of the astute yet kind Robert Finley. Many thanks to my classmates, close friends, and a few hardy souls who took the time to read and critique my work. Moyra Buchan, Ginny Ryan, Donna Ball, and Titia Praamsma, your thoughtful remarks have strengthened both the final version, and my backbone.

Writers NL, for their exceptionally good programming and support, especially the manuscript evaluation service, which helped me to get good advice from Jenny Higgins. And thanks to Larry Matthews, who encouraged me to submit to Breakwater when I was having doubts.

And finally everyone at Breakwater Books: Rebecca Rose, substantive editor Shelley Egan, copy editor Marianne Ward, Carola Kern, Norma Noseworthy, Jocelyne Thomas, Beth Oberholtzer, Rebecca Roberts, Emma Cole, and Bashir Behrawan.

I can be reached through my website if you would like to offer any comments on the subject of this book. I look forward to hearing from you.

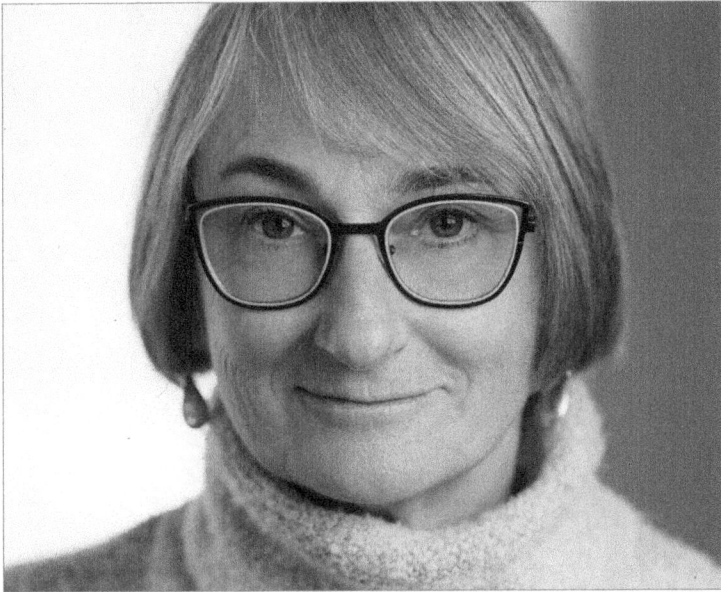

Debbie McGee made her first film in Vancouver in 1983, and her last film in St. John's in 2013. In between those markers, she worked as a writer and director of short dramas and NFB documentaries before joining the Media Unit at Memorial University of Newfoundland and Labrador as Producer/Director. She has been an active volunteer with arts organizations throughout her career, serving on many boards, juries, and councils. Debbie is a mother and a grandmother. She lives in St. John's, Newfoundland, with her adorable puppy Cammie.

Her films and awards are available for viewing on her website: debbiemcgee.ca.